SRN REVIEW BOOK
OBJECTIVE TEST QUESTIONS
FOR STUDENT NURSES

Edited and Compiled by
LYNN COPCUTT SRN DN(London) RNT. Cert.Ed.
Senior Tutor, Queen Elizabeth School of Nursing,
Edgbaston, Birmingham.

PASTEST SERVICE
Hemel Hempstead
Hertfordshire England

© 1981 PASTEST SERVICE,
P.O. Box 81, Hemel Hempstead, Hertfordshire

First published 1981
Reprinted 1981
ISBN 0 906896 01 0

| **British Library Cataloguing in Publication Data** |
| Copcutt, Lynn |
| SRN review book. |
| 1. Medicine — Problems, exercises, etc. |
| I. Title |
| 610'.76   RT65 |
| ISBN 0 906896 01 0 |

Phototypeset by ADS, 72 Sackville Street, Manchester.
Printed by Hazell, Watson and Viney Limited, Aylesbury.

CONTENTS

Brackets indicate the number of questions in each subject.
Total number of questions 240.

NOTES TO THE READER

This book has been produced to assist student nurses preparing for the multiple choice paper of the State Final Examination for the General Register, established by the General Nursing Council for England and Wales.

All examinations create anxiety for candidates. Multiple choice questions can pose particular difficulties for some people because of lack of experience in attempting this type of test; or because previously they have been faced with questions which bear little similarity to those found in the actual examination. I therefore feel there is a need for this book and its sister edition for pupil nurses, because they contain carefully selected, pretested and validated questions.

Practising nurse teachers were invited to submit questions for consideration. Over 2,000 questions were scrutinized to obtain the 240 finally accepted. After initial editing, the questions were compiled into test papers of 60 questions each. These tests were then taken by a minimum of 100 finalist student nurses in more than 60 schools of nursing throughout the country.

Computer analysis followed and only those questions meeting predetermined levels of difficulty and discrimination were considered for inclusion. Additionally, comments received from student nurses and teaching staff participating with the pre-testing of questions were considered. Thank you all for your co-operation.

The preparation of multiple choice tests is not easy, but every attempt has been made to ensure that this publication will become a helpful part of the arduous task of examination revision.

This book contains 240 multiple choice questions, of which 180 are subdivided into the 13 main subject areas of the final examination, according to the specification grid of the GNC. The last 60 questions are grouped together as a practice examination and have been compiled to cover the range of topics and degree of difficulty the student is likely to meet.

Each question consists of an initial statement followed by four alternative answers, marked A B C D. Only *one* of these is correct.

Questions are printed on the right-hand page, with the correct answers and explanations on the following page. Alongside each answer, you will find a percentage figure which indicates the number of finalist nurses who chose the correct answer during pre-testing of the questions. Questions with a high percentage are easier than those with a low percentage. By using this information, you will be able to identify areas which need concentrated revison. It will also enable you to assess your own level of performance relative to that of other finalists. Attempt each question before you look at the answers, this is the best way to test your knowledge and highlight strengths and weaknesses.

Finally, a word of thanks to the many people who have assisted with the preparation of this book, especially Shirley Low and the staff of the General Nursing Council's Examinations and Assessment Department without whose help the publication of this book would not have been possible. I am most grateful to you all.

L.C.

REVISION GUIDE

The following checklist is intended to help you structure and plan your revision effectively, although the list is by no means complete.

Try to adopt a "total care" approach using the following master plan: it can be applied to any patient care situation and encompasses both drug therapy and nursing observations, as well as community and hospital based management.

Relate physiology to the signs and symptoms as you work through each list of disorders, rather than try to master each independently.

MASTER PLAN
Identify patient problems and the measures needed to relieve or prevent them in relation to:
a) Social needs
b) Psychological Needs
c) Physical needs:-

> Mobility
> Nutrition
> Elimination
> Hygiene
> Comfort/relief of pain
> Respiration
> Wound
> Safety (include First Aid)
> Prevention of complications

CHECK LIST
1. *Professional responsibilities*

> e.g. Ward emergenices
> Dealing with enquiries
> Junior nurses
> Confidentiality
> Channels of communication
> Functions of the GNC (to be replaced by Central Council after 1982)
> Complaints procedure
> The role of Health Visitors/Midwives
> The role of Community Health Councils
> Awareness of well-known nursing research

5. *Excretion*

  e.g. Investigations of renal/genito-urinary tract
    Causes of haematuria
    Reasons for nephrectomy
    Infections of kidney
    Infections of bladder
    Incontinence of urine
    Retention of urine
    Acute renal failure
    Nephrotic syndrome
    Chronic renal failure
    Prostate gland disorders
    Tumours of bladder: benign/malignant
    Renal colic/calculi
    Water and electrolyte balance

6. *Circulation*

  e.g. Investigations of circulatory system
    Blood groups, X-matching, transfusion
    Anaemia
    Haemorrhage
    Leukaemia
    Angina pectoris
    Myocardial infarction
    Heart failure
    Valve stenosis/incompetence
    Subacute bacterial endocarditis
    Oedema
    Hypertension
    Varicose veins/haemorrhoids
    Lymphatic disorders
    Circulatory deficiency
    Blood clotting disorders
    Shock

7. *Neurology*

   e.g. Epilepsy
        Subarachnoid haemorrhage
        Cerebrovascular accident
        Unconsciousness
        Meningitis
        Multiple Sclerosis
        Pain
        Head Injury
        Types/causes/effects of paralysis
        Investigations of neurological disorders
        Cataracts
        Glaucoma
        Corneal abrasions
        Blindness
        Deafness
        Tonsillectomy
        Tracheostomy
        Laryngectomy
        Otitis Media

8. *Hormonal Control*

   e.g. Myxoedema
        Thyrotoxicosis
        Partial Thyroidectomy
        Diabetes Mellitus
        Diabetes Insipidus
        Underactivity of Adrenal glands
        Overactivity of Adrenal glands
        Physiological effects of hormones
        Cushing's syndrome
        Investigations of endocrine dysfunction

9. *Locomotion*

   e.g. Rheumatoid Arthritis
        Osteoarthritis
        Low back pain
        Limb amputation
        Fractures : Potts
                Colles
                Neck of femur
                Shaft of femur
                Tibia/fibula
                Pelvis
                Ribs
      Bone healing

10. *Reproduction*
    e.g. Menstruation and menstrual disorders
    Infertility
    Ectopic pregnancy
    Outline normal pregnancy/delivery
    Abortion
    Uterine fibroids
         prolapse
         malignancy
    Veneral diseases
    Breast disorders

11. *Immune response*
    e.g. Immunity/Immunisation
    Auto immune disorders
    Allergies/Anaphylaxis
    Communicable diseases : Measles
                            German Measles
                            Poliomyelitis
                            Tetanus
                            Chickenpox
                            Mumps

12. *The Skin*
    e.g. Burns
    Scalds
    Eczema
    Psoriasis
    Scabies
    Fungal infections
    Herpes
    Wound healing
    Pressure sores
    Pilonidal sinus

13. *Drugs and Therapeutic Hazards*
    e.g. Legislative control
    Infusions
    Transfusions
    Steroids
    Antibiotics
    Anticoagulants
    Analgesics
    Miotics
    Mydriatics
    Diuretics
    Insulin

PROFESSIONAL RESPONSIBILITIES

1. **Which of the following make up the Primary Health Care Team:**

   A   GP, Health Visitor, Home Help, Occupational Therapist
   B   Social Worker, Physiotherapist, Occupational Therapist,
       District Nursing Sister
   C   Midwifery Sister, District Nursing Sister, GP, Health Visitor
   D   District Nursing Sister, Social Worker, Home Help, Health
       Visitor

2. **The meals on wheels service is the responsibility of the**

   A   Primary Health Care Team
   B   Social Service Department
   C   Area Health Authority
   D   Geriatric Community Service

3. **In case of fire on the ward, the nurse should first of all**

   A   evacuate the patients
   B   raise the fire alarm
   C   close the doors and windows
   D   reassure the patients

4. **The Health visitor is responsible for the welfare of a baby from
   the age of**

   A   48 hours
   B   5 days
   C   10 days
   D   15 days

5. **You are on duty in a small ward at night when a strange adult
   enters the ward. He threatens you with a knife and demands that
   you give him the morphine from the drug cupboard. Should you**

   A   give him the drugs then call the police as soon as he has left
       the ward
   B   under no circumstances give him the drugs
   C   try to talk him out of it and explain that there is no morphine
       in the cupboard anyway
   D   tell him you will go and get some morphine the gently slip out
       of the ward and try to summon help

Answers overleaf

1. C   79%

The Primary Health Care Team consists of the Midwifery Sister, District Nursing Sister, GP, and Health Visitor.

2. B   86%

A C and D provide health care. The Social Services Department is responsible for the provision of meals on wheels which is not categorised as health care.

3. B   90%

Once the fire alarm has been sounded, other people will be available to assist with all the other tasks. It is vital that there is minimal delay in alerting the fire brigade.

4. C   77%

The Health Visitor is responsible for the welfare of all children both normal and handicapped, in the 0-5 years age range, at home and in clinics. She is also involved with hospital liaison, health education and controlling infectious diseases. Additionally the Health Visitor plays an important role in the prevention and early detection of ill health in the elderly and in the screening of members of the public of all ages in clinics. The Health Visitor is a State Registered Nurse who must also hold the Health Visitors Certificate awarded by the Council for the Education and Training of Health Visitors.

5. A   41%

As the stranger has threatened violence, steps must be taken to avoid harm to the nurse. The police must be informed as a theft has technically occurred.

6. **Which of the following is the correct membership of the District Management Team:**

   A District Community   C District Personnel Officer
           Physician   District Finance Officer
           District Nursing Officer   District Administrator
           District Finance Officer   Director of Nurse Education
           District Administrator   D Consultant Physician
   B District Finance Officer   District Nursing Officer
           Divisional Nursing Officer   District Administrator
           General Practitioner   District Personnel Officer
           Senior Nursing Officer

7. **As a nurse in charge, you are trying to cope with an incident on the ward where a male patient is being violent. A senior nursing officer appears on the ward to do a ward round. Should you**

   A ignore the SNO and get on with the urgent job at hand
   B send a junior nurse to look after the SNO
   C enlist the SNO's aid in dealing with the violent patient
   D ask the SNO to get some male nurses quickly

8. **A patient is being resuscitated following a cardiac arrest. A junior nurse on duty has not seen this procedure before. Should she**

   A be exchanged with a more senior nurse from another ward
   B attend to other patients and learn about the procedure later
   C help with the procedure and discuss it afterwards
   D attend to other patients whilst observing the procedure at intervals

9. **One function of Community Health Councils is to**

   A control community voluntary services
   B act as a public watchdog
   C carry out health education in inner cities
   D regulate local authority health spending

10. **Which of the following are eligible for free dental treatment:**

    A university students
    B old age pensioners
    C expectant mothers
    D physically disabled

Answers overleaf

6. A 50%

Following reorganisation in 1974, these officials were appointed as the paid member of the District Management Team.

7. C 61%

The more experienced nurse should use such experience to deal with the patient. Other tasks including the ward round, are secondary to this situation.

8. C 49%

A cardiac arrest can be a stressful situation for a junior nurse. She should have the opportunity to participate in the situation and discuss it afterwards so she is more able to cope next time such an event occurs.

9. B 45%

Community Health Councils were set up in 1974 in order to help safeguard public interest in all aspects of health care provision. They comment or advise on many aspects of the work of the NHS and act as a public watchdog.

10. C 90%

The Department of Health and Social Security exempt expectant mothers from dental charges. The other groups mentioned must pay a proportion of such charges.

THE PHYSIOLOGICAL AND PSYCHOLOGICAL NEEDS OF THE INDIVIDUAL

11. **The anterior fontanelle closes within**

    A 6 weeks of life
    B 9 months of life
    C 18 months of life
    D 2 years of life

alculation of Basal Metabolic Rate estimates the

    A calorific requirements related to body weight
    B relationship between pulse and blood pressure at rest
    C cardiac output in relation to prolonged activity
    D oxygen used whilst resting for a specific time

13. **A child is admitted to the Paediatric Ward clutching a small grubby torn blanket. Should you**

    A give the blanket to the mother to take home
    B let the child keep it by her
    C wash the blanket in disinfectant
    D put the blanket out of reach but not out of sight

14. **Which of the following periods refers to the first month of life:**

    A pre-natal
    B peri-natal
    C neo-natal
    D foetal

15. **Which one of the following is thought to be *most* important when trying to increase a person's motivation:**

    A always reward whether goal is achieved or not
    B only reward when perfection is finally reached
    C aim to over-motivate rather than under-motivate
    D make sure their goals are achievable

Answers overleaf

11. C 37%

Closing of the fontanelles is one of the normal milestones of early life.
The anterior fontanelle should close by eighteen months.

12. D 69%

Used to aid diagnosis, changes in metabolic rate can be measured. In thyrotoxicosis for example, the BMR is raised because of the effects of thyroxine.

13. B 87%

Anything which represents security to a small child on admission to hospital must be retained by the child at all times — whatever it's condition.

14. C 74%

Neo-natal refers to the first month of life. Hence, neo-natal mortality is the death rate occurring during the first months of life as compared with the remaining 11 months of the first year.

15. D 82%

Realistic goals are essential for suitable motivation. If the goals are seen to be unattainable, then no effort will be made to try and achieve them.

16. **In order to re-establish a patient's mobility as quickly as possible following a stroke, the *most* important action is to**

    A   position the limb correctly
    B   perform passive limb exercises
    C   turn the patient 2 hourly
    D   apply splints to the affected limbs

17. **Impairment to the sense of smell**

    A   typically follows thalmic damage
    B   generally accompanies the ageing process
    C   is typically an early sign of occipital lobe tumour
    D   is always linked with an impairment in the sense of taste

18. **A patient recovering from depression is considered by the doctor to be fit for weekend leave. It is *most* important to advise his wife**

    A   of the suicide risk
    B   to note husband's mood and behaviour
    C   to enjoy the weekend
    D   to return husband safely on time

19. **Blood pressure is maintained as a result of**

    A   blood viscosity, cardiac output and constriction of arterioles
    B   venous pressure, stroke volume and constriction of arterioles
    C   venous pressure, stroke volume and constriction of capillaries
    D   blood viscosity, cardiac output and constriction of capillaries

20. **A normal healthy baby will double its birth weight by the age of**

    A   three months
    B   six months
    C   nine months
    D   twelve months

Answers overleaf

16.   B   76%

Passive limb movements help to reduce joint stiffness. Adequate joint movement is essential if mobility is to be regained.

17.   B   83%

Nerve cells and thus the areas they supply degenerate with age. Smell is no exception to this.

18.   B   57%

Observation of the patient's mood and behaviour away from hospital is significant in assessing the patient's readiness for discharge.

19.   A   65%

In order to maintain blood pressure it is essential that there is an adequate amount of blood circulating. Cardiac output is the amount of blood leaving the heart per minute. The thicker or more viscous the blood, the higher the systolic pressure needed in order to propel it around the arteries. Finally, the resistance in the arterioles is governed by their diameter. The narrower the lumen, the greater the peripheral resistance and the higher the pressure.

20.   B   43%

Weight gain of this order is one of the milestones of normal physical development.

21. **The term "cor pulmonale" may be defined as**

    A   disease of the heart or pulmonary vessels, secondary to right-sided heart failure
    B   left-sided heart failure secondary to disease of the lungs or pulmonary vessels
    C   left-sided heart failure secondary to right sided heart failure
    D   right-sided heart failure secondary to disease of the lungs or pulmonary vessels

22. **Which of the following is increased when a patient has severe emphysema:**

    A   tidal volume
    B   inspiratory reserve
    C   vital capacity
    D   residual volume

23. **Which one of the following characteristics would best describe the sputum of a patient suffering from lobar pneumonia:**

    A   frothy
    B   purulent
    C   rusty
    D   mucoid

24. **A "barrel chest" is mainly due to**

    A   lack of nerve impulses
    B   increase in residual air
    C   hypertrophy of muscle
    D   abnormality of blood gases

25. **Paroxysmal nocturnal dyspnoea results from**

    A   pulmonary valve stenosis
    B   right ventricular failure
    C   bronchitis with emphysema
    D   left ventricular failure

Answers overleaf

9

21. D 66%

Cor pulmonale is heart disease following on from chronic lung disease which strains the right ventricle.

22. D 67%

Emphysema is a condition of the lungs where there is distension of the alveoli and loss of the division between the alveoli. The alveoli walls become thin and eventually break down, and the lungs lose their normal elasticity and become over-distended. Due to the over-distension, the residual volume of air in the lungs is increased. The residual volume is the amount of air left in the respiratory passages after expiration. Tidal volume is the amount of air breathed in and out during quiet respiration. Inspiratory reserve or capacity is the amount of air we can breathe in forcefully. The vital capacity is the largest volume of air breathed out after the deepest inspiration.

23. C 43%

Rusty coloured sputum, due to the presence of blood in it, is a feature of lobar pneumonia. Destroyed red cells pass through the damaged alveolar walls into the alveoli as a result of the inflammatory process.

24. B 45%

Barrel chest, sometimes a feature of emphysema, results from lack of elastic recoil in the chest. The effect of this is to lead to an increase in residual air.

25. D 67%

Paroxysmal nocturnal dyspnoea, also known as cardiac asthma, occurs when the patient adopts a more recumbant posture, usually at night, often waking the patient. Venous return to the heart is improved, but because of the heart failure, the respiratory congestion is worsened.

26. **Atelectasis is:**

   A   collapse of the alveoli supplied by obstructed bronchioles
   B   a rise of the intrapleural pressure on one side
   C   an increase in the physiological dead space
   D   vasodilatation in the alveoli supplied by obstructed
       bronchioles

27. **Which of the following anatomical features in the bronchiole will cause bronchospasm:**

   A   bands of fibro-cartilage
   B   smooth muscle layers
   C   ciliated epithelial tissue
   D   fibro-elastic tissue

28. **Which of the following defines the vital capacity of the lungs:**

   A   the maximum volume of air that can be expelled from the
       lungs after breathing in deeply
   B   the volume of air remaining in the lungs after expiring as
       much as possible
   C   the minimum volume of air needed with each breath to
       maintain life
   D   the difference is volume between a normal breath and the
       maximum possible breath.

29. **After some years, chronic bronchitis may affect the heart by causing initially**

   A   left ventricular failure
   B   right ventricular failure
   C   angina pectoris
   D   myocardial ischaemia

30. **The primary purpose of giving oxygen to a patient is to**

   A   encourage deep breathing
   B   maintain tissue cell function
   C   relieve airway obstruction
   D   relieve apprehension

Answers overleaf

11

26.   **A**   **72%**

Obstruction of part of the bronchial tree can result from an inhaled foreign body, a plug of mucus or a tumour. The blockage causes a condition known as ATELECTASIS which is incomplete expansion of part of the lung due to the blockage. The air in the part of the lung beyond the blockage is absorbed into the blood stream and is not replaced so that the affected alveoli collapse.

27.   **B**   **76%**

Spasm can only occur in muscle, thus in bronchospasm it must be the smooth muscle layers which are affected.

28.   **A**   **56%**

Vital capacity is measured by the subject inspiring as much air as possible in one breath and then expiring it fully. The average measurement in the male is 4.5 litres.

29.   **B**   **37%**

Any chronic lung condition will strain the right side of the heart, leading to failure. Gradually, the left side of the heart also becomes involved and left ventricular failure results too.

30.   **B**   **81%**

Without an adequate oxygen supply, cells will die. The primary purpose of oxygen administration is the maintenance of tissue cell function.

31. **Oxygen diffuses from the alveoli to the capillaries because the**

    A oxygen pressure is higher in the capillaries
    B alveolar pressure is raised
    C oxygen pressure is lower in the capillaries
    D level of carbon dioxide is higher in the capillaries

32. **Which one of the following affects the rate and depth of respirations when a patient has pneumonia:**

    A fibrosed lung tissue
    B pain on inhalation
    C spasm of the terminal bronchioles
    D distension of the alveoli

33. **A patient who has a pleural effusion feels breathless because**

    A fluid is accumulating in the lung
    B there is pressure on the lung
    C the diaphragm is irritated
    D the diaphragmatic movement is increased

34. **Patients suffering from a common cold may lose their appreciation of food because**

    A there is impairment of the sense of smell
    B they have difficulty in swallowing due to blocked nasal
        passages
    C viral infections always affect the appetite
    D nausea and vomiting lead to anorexia

35. **A patient has an exacerbation of chronic bronchitis. Which of the following treatments should be discouraged:**

    A intravenous aminophylline
    B oxygen via a polymask
    C Mucodyne syrup
    D Salbutamol inhaler

Answers overleaf

31. C 46%

Diffusion is the process whereby gases and liquids intermingle when brought into contact until the density is equal throughout. Therefore, there is diffusion of some of the substances from an area of high pressure to one of low pressure. Oxygen concentration is lower in the alveolar capillaries than the alveoli themselves, so oxygen diffuses into them.

32. B 49%

The pleura over the affected lobe of the lung is irritated leading to pleurisy. Such irritation leads to the typical pleuritic pain on inspiration, when the lungs expand and the pleura are stretched.

33. B 84%

An effusion is the leakage of fluid into a body cavity due to congestion or inflammation. In the case of a pleural effusion, the fluid has accumulated outside the lungs in the pleural cavity. The pleural effusion causes pressure on the lungs due to the increasing fluid levels. The patient complains of breathlessness and the respiratory rate is often increased to help compensate for the decreased respiratory area.

34. A 84%

A common cold is defined as an inflamed state of mucous membrane especially of the nose and throat. The nerve endings of the sense of smell (from the 1st cranial nerve, the olfactory nerve) are situated in the highest part of the nasal cavity. Patients lose their appreciation of food as their sense of smell is impaired due to the local inflammation around the nerve ending. Patients may be disinclined to eat due to nasal congestion but this does not alter appreciation of food unless the nerve endings are affected. Viral infections can take many forms in the body and may be totally unrelated to the appetite. The common cold does not usually produce nausea or vomiting.

35. B 70%

A polymask gives a high concentration of oxygen. In health, the respiratory centre responds to carbon dioxide concentration in the blood. In chronic bronchitis, carbon dioxide levels in the blood are raised at all times, making the respiratory centre insensitive to it. If too much oxygen is given, respiration slows and eventually stops.

DIGESTION

36. **Spider naevi are a characteristic of**

    A   vitamin C deficiency
    B   overdosage with anticoagulants
    C   cirrhosis of the liver
    D   haemophilia

37. **Which of the following is a partially digested form of food:**

    A   amino acids
    B   fatty acids
    C   glucose
    D   lactose

38. **Prior to partial gastrectomy a patient should have the full details of post-operative care explained to him. The *most* important advantage of this is**

    A   confidence in hospital staff is heightened
    B   undue anxiety and worry is eliminated
    C   co-operation and recovery rate are increased
    D   progress can be assessed by the patient

39. **The absorption of vitamin K from the intestine requires the presence of**

    A   enterokinase
    B   bile salts
    C   pancreozymin
    D   secretin

40. **Which of the following suggest carcinoma of the rectum:**

    A   diarrhoea and passage of blood via the rectum
    B   change of bowel habits plus bleeding via the rectum
    C   constipation plus bleeding via the rectum
    D   difficulty in micturition plus passage of blood via the rectum

Answers overleaf

15

36. C   73%

Spider naevi occurs in cirrhosis. They are fine-branching arterioles radiating and coalescing into a web of purple-red discolouration.

37. D   41%

Of the alternatives given LACTOSE is the only partially digested food. Amino acids are the digested form of protein, fatty acids and glycerol are the end products of fat digestion, and glucose is a simple monosaccharide easily absorbed into the blood. Lactose requires further digestion by LACTASE before it can be absorbed by the intestinal villi.

38. C   68%

If the patient understands his post-operative care then he is more likely to co-operate with staff, thus minimising risks of complications and facilitating his recovery. Whilst the other options could apply, C is the most important.

39. B   64%

Vitamin K is fat soluble. If fat is not being digested with the aid of bile salts, then vitamin K cannot be absorbed. Steatorrhoea will result and the stool will contain undigested fats and all the ingested vitamin K.

40. B   62%

Of the alternatives given, a change in bowel habits accompanied by the passage of frank blood is most suggestive of carcinoma of the rectum. Proctoscopy, sigmoidoscopy and biopsy will confirm the diagnosis.

41. **When muscle tissues are broken down, they form a protein called**

    A   urea
    B   uric acid
    C   creatinine
    D   amino acid

42. **Which one of the following is a function of the gall bladder:**

    A   production of bile
    B   concentration of bile
    C   absorption of bile
    D   secretion of bile

43. **Diarrhoea is most likely to result from**

    A   antibiotic therapy
    B   diverticulosis
    C   faecal incontinence
    D   escherichia coli

44. **A patient is to undergo emergency surgery at 7 pm because of intestinal obstruction. His wife is with him on admission and should be told to**

    A   return home and visit later that evening
    B   return home and telephone later
    C   stay by her husband as long as she wishes
    D   stay until surgery is completed if she wishes

45. **Diverticulosis occurs in the colon as a result of**

    A   thickening of the wall of the large bowel
    B   weakening of the wall of the large bowel
    C   a diet high in cellulose fibre
    D   a diet containing little meat

Answers overleaf

41. C 40%

Creatinine is the waste product of muscle tissue breakdown. It is excreted, unaltered, via the kidney.

42. B 47%

One of the functions of the gall bladder is to concentrate bile. Bile is manufactured by the liver and is then stored in the gall bladder. During this time, some of the water is re-absorbed by the gall bladder, concentrating the bile.

43. A 63%

Patients receiving antibiotic therapy may develop diarrhoea because of the adverse effect of the drug on the normal flora of the bowel. This enables pathogens not sensitive to the drug to flourish, and diarrhoea results.

44. D 73%

The patient's wife should initially be invited to stay until the operation is completed; if she needs to return home for domestic reasons then options A or B could be suggested. Option C is impractical as the patient needs emergency surgery.

45. B 69%

Diverticulosis of the colon is due to a weakening of the gut wall. (It may also be caused by increased intra-luminal pressure.) As a result of the weakness, pockets or pouches of mucosa are formed. If these pouches then become inflamed, diverticulitis has developed with the risk of subsequent perforation.

46.   The term renal threshold indicates the

    A   amount of urine the kidneys can produce
    B   amount of a substance the kidneys can reabsorb
    C   ability of the kidney to excrete sodium
    D   ability of the kidneys to concentrate urine

47.   Excessive vomiting is known as

    A   hyperhidrosis
    B   hyperemesis
    C   hypermotility
    D   hyperphagia

48.   The commonest organism causing urinary tract infection is

    A   escherichia coli
    B   streptococcus viridans
    C   clostridium welchii
    D   staphylococcus aureus

49.   Following nephrectomy the patient has one normally functioning kidney. The urinary output would therefore be reduced by

    A   0%
    B   25%
    C   50%
    D   75%

50.   In the initial stages of acute glomerular nephritis, the diet should contain

    A   free fluids only
    B   restricted fluids only
    C   free fluids and 120 gm. protein
    D   restricted fluids and 40 gm. protein

Answers overleaf

46.   B   54%

The term 'threshold' indicates tolerance of a structure, in this case the tolerance or amount of substance which can be reabsorbed by the kidney.

47.   B   84%

Excessive vomiting is known as hyperemesis. The prefix hyper means above or too much.
Hyperhidrosis — excessive perspiration
Hypermotility — excessive action
Hyperphagia — overeating

48.   A   70%

Escherichia coli is a normal inhabitant of the bowel. It is thus quite easy for it to pass to the urinary tract, especially in women, and cause ascending infection. Clostridium welchii normally resides in the soil, streptococcus viridans in the throat and staphylococcus aureus in the nose.

49.   A   85%

Following nephrectomy, the remaining kidney takes over the entire urine output. Urinary output must remain as it was when both kidneys were functioning, providing, of course, that other influencing factors remain the same.

50.   D   59%

Treatment of acute glomerular nephritis aims to maintain water and electrolyte balance but restrict protein intake until spontaneous recovery of renal function returns.

51. Serum acid phosphatase levels are useful in the diagnosis of

A diabetic ketosis
B hyperkalaemia
C carcinoma of prostate
D syphilis

52. On which part of the nephron does the antidiuretic hormone act:

A bowmans capsule
B loop of henle
C proximal tubule
D distal tubule

53. Which of the following would be responsible for the hypertension of renal impairment:

A antidiuretic hormone
B urea
C cholesterol
D renin

54. In non-obstructive carcinoma of the prostate, the treatment of choice is

A suprapubic prostatectomy
B transurethral prostatectomy
C retropubic prostatectomy
D oestrogen therapy

55. In nephrotic syndrome the

A tubule cells can no longer reabsorb sufficient water
B glomeruli permit leakage of plasma proteins
C glomeruli can no longer filter water and urea
D tubule cells leak plasma protein into the filtrate

Answers overleaf

51.   C   55%

Serum acid phosphatase is always raised in carcinoma of the prostate. However, care must be taken that blood for acid phosphatase is taken before the prostate is palpated, because during rectal examination the level rises.

52.   D   46%

The antidiuretic hormone acts upon the distal tubule (and the collecting tubule) regulating the reabsorption of water from the filtrate.

53.   D   43%

Renin is secreted by the kidney. Although its action is not fully understood, it is believed to be a hypertensive agent. Renin acts upon angiotensinogen in the plasma to produce angiotensin. This angiotensin then influences the production of aldosterone. As a result, more sodium is reabsorbed in the tubule of the kidney.

54.   D   55%

Carcinoma of the prostate is difficult to remove surgically and if no obstruction is present, surgery is not indicated. Hormone therapy is very effective in reducing the size of the prostate gland, and is effective against its tendency to metastasise.

55.   B   48%

In nephrotic syndrome (nephrosis), the protein content of the blood is lost due to damage to the glomerulus. Albumin (a plasma protein responsible for maintaining the osmotic pressure of the blood) is lost in the urine and oedema is inevitable. The albumin must be replaced, as this is the substance of which all cell cytoplasm is made, and so a high protein diet is given in nephrotic syndrome.

56. **Excessive albuminuria causes**

   A   dehydration
   B   bruising
   C   infection
   D   oedema

57. **Which one of the following is most important when nursing a patient with acute glomerular nephritis:**

   A   bed rest and warmth
   B   high fluid intake
   C   high protein diet
   D   analgesia and sedation

58. **Which one of the following investigations is most useful in diagnosing carcinoma of the kidney:**

   A   urea and electrolytes
   B   retrograde pyelogram
   C   renal arteriogram
   D   electrophoresis

59. **Following a nephrectomy fluids are restricted because**

   A   parenteral fluids are given
   B   paralytic ileus could develop
   C   oliguria occurs post-operatively
   D   retention of urine is likely

60. **Filtration occurs in the nephron because of**

   A   glomerular damage
   B   raised osmotic pressure
   C   adequate systolic pressure
   D   raised urea levels

Answers overleaf

56. D 62%

Albumin is one of the plasma proteins; if it is lost the osmotic pressure in the circulation is reduced, thus allowing fluid to leave the circulation and enter tissue spaces. This fluid is known as oedema.

57. A 40%

One of the aims in treating this condition is to ensure rest and warmth as the patient is ill, oliguric and oedematous. Protein and fluids would be restricted.

58. C 50%

The malignant renal tissue will have an increased blood supply which will be demonstrated by a renal arteriogram.

59. B 80%

Following a nephrectomy fluids are restricted until bowel sounds return, as, after any abdominal surgery, a paralytic ileus may develop. If excessive oral fluids are given, vomiting will result.

60. C 77%

The kidney needs an adequate blood supply in order for filtration to occur, systolic pressure is therefore important. Prolonged hypotension will result in oliguria, as renal function is impaired.

61. On walking 100 yards, a man has calf pain which disappears at rest. This is most likely to be caused by

A   Buerger's disease
B   deep vein thrombosis
C   pressure upon the sciatic nerve
D   varicose veins

62. A patient suffering from hypertension is likely to be prescribed

A   analgesia and hypnotics
B   diuretics and analgesia
C   barbiturates and tranquillisers
D   diuretics and tranquillisers

63. When the ventricles of the heart contract, which of the following occurs:

A   mitral valve and aortic valve open
B   aortic and pulmonary valves open
C   tricuspid and pulmonary valves open
D   tricuspid and aortic valves open

64. The P wave of the normal electrocardiogram is caused by

A   conduction of the bundle of His
B   ventricular systole
C   artrial wall conduction
D   ventricular diastole

65. Hypochromic microcytic anaemia results from an inadequacy of

A   folate
B   iron
C B_{12}
D   protein

61.   A   65%

In Buerger's disease, the smaller peripheral arteries with the associated veins and nerves are involved in a fibrotic process which results in peripheral ischaemia. This leads to a condition of intermittent claudication when insufficient blood reaches the leg veins on excercise. As the condition deteriorates, the patient experiences calf pain even at rest. However, in the early stages of the disease, the calf pain appears on exercise and disappears at rest when blood is able to circulate sufficiently to the legs. The other conditions cause pain in the legs but the pain is not relieved by rest.

62.   D   75%

Diuretics exert a substantial antihypertensive action and in mild cases of hypertension are often the only drugs required. Tranquillisers allay anxiety and have a calming effect on the patient. The phenothiazines and related drugs intensify the effects of sympathetic nerve stimulation, which accounts for the vasodilation and hypotensive effects.

63.   B   88%

The atria contract together and force blood through the bicuspid and tricuspid valves into the ventricles. When the ventricles contract, the bicuspid and tricuspid valves close and blood is pumped out through the open aortic valve and pulmonary valve into the aorta and pulmonary artery respectively.

64.   C   33%

The P wave is produced by the spread of the impulse from the sino-atrial node over the atrial muscle, causing depolorisation of the atria. This is then recorded by the electrocardiogram.

65.   B   75%

When iron is lacking in the body, haemoglobin cannot be made in the right quantity and the red blood cells become small (microcytic) and pale (hypochromic).

66. **Bacterial endocarditis is most likely to be due to the**

    A   pneumococcus
    B   treponema pallidum
    C   streptococcus viridans
    D   staphylococcus aureus

67. **Distended neck veins are usually a sign of**

    A   left ventricular failure
    B   right ventricular failure
    C   mitral stenosis
    D   mitral incompetence

68. **Which of the following complications is likely to accompany pernicious anaemia:**

    A   peptic ulceration
    B   carcinoma of the stomach
    C   chronic renal failure
    D   heart failure

69. **The site usually chosen for bone marrow puncture in a child is the**

    A   fibula
    B   sternum
    C   femur
    D   tibia

70. **Which one of the following actions will help return the pH of the blood of an acidotic patient to normal:**

    A   hyperventilation
    B   hypoventilation
    C   apnoea
    D   orthopnoea

Answers overleaf

66. C 69%

Streptococcus viridans is a normal commensal of the throat that may enter the blood stream and can settle on diseased heart valves causing sub-acute bacterial endocarditis.

67. B 75%

The distension of the jugular veins in the neck are due to congestion of the veins. The congestion is a result of blood being unable to enter the right atria via the superior vena cava in sufficient quantity, because the right ventricle is not functioning adequately. Mitral stenosis, mitral incompetence and left ventricular failure all cause problems on the left side of the heart and it is the pulmonary circulation which becomes congested.

68. D 45%

Pernicious anaemia primarily results from atrophy of the stomach which fails to secrete normal gastric juices. A result of the failure of gastric function is the failure of absorption of vitamin B_{12} from the food due to the deficiency of the Intrinsic factor. There is also achlorhydria. When vitamin B_{12} is lacking, the bone marrow cannot produce enough red blood cell envelopes, although there is enough haemoglobin. If the anaemia is severe, the prolonged tachycardia may lead to heart failure.

69. D 57%

The tibial plateau is the site most usually chosen for bone marrow puncture in the child. Generally the sternum is too thin and there is danger of perforation.

70. A 70%

In the acidotic patient, hyperventilation will lower the carbon dioxide level in the blood, reducing the acidosis and therefore raising the pH.

71. **Which one of the following is the most likely complication of myocardial infarction:**

A renal failure
B cerebral haemorrhage
C left ventricular failure
D pulmonary embolism

72. **The oedema of congestive cardiac failure is due to**

A raised arterial pressure
B raised venous pressure
C lowered arterial pressure
D lowered venous pressure

73. **Agglutination is likely to occur when blood group**

A O is given to A
B AB is given to B
C A is given to AB
D O is given to B

74. **The most common clinical feature of thrombophlebitis in the lower limb is**

A cyanosis of the affected limb
B pain in the calf of the leg
C oedema of the ankle
D dilatation of the veins

75. **In haemolytic anaemia there is**

A a cessation in the blood-forming factors
B decrease in red cell formation
C chronic blood loss
D excessive destruction of red blood cells

Answers overleaf

71. C   56%

The infarction puts a strain on the myocardium and often makes it inefficient. The left ventricular myocardium will attempt to compensate for the reduced cardiac output by enlarging. Eventual failure may result when the hypertrophied muscle can no longer maintain cardiac output satisfactorily.

72. B   59%

A common sign in congestive cardiac failure is a jugular venous pulse, an invariable sign of raised venous pressure which leads to oedema. So far as the arterial pressure is concerned, neither hypotension (as in shock) nor hypertension are characterised by oedema.

73. B   80%

Group AB has agglutinogens A and B present in red cells. Group B has agglutinins A in the plasma. When agglutinin A contacts agglutinogen A, then agglutination will result.

74. B   66%

Pain or tenderness in the calf of the leg is the most common clinical feature of thrombo-phlebitis and should be reported immediately.

75. D   84%

Haemolysis means breakdown of red blood cells. If this occurs excessively for any reason, then anaemia will result. Therefore, in haemolytic anaemia, there is excessive destruction of red cells.

76. **When the mitral valves close, there is a rise in pressure within the**

   A   right atrium, above that in the right ventricle
   B   right ventricle, above that in the right atrium
   C   left ventricle, above that in the left atrium
   D   left atrium, above that in the left ventricle

77. **When blood clots, the soluble substance which becomes insoluble is**

   A   fibrinogen
   B   prothrombin
   C   calcium ions
   D   thrombin

78. **In left ventricular failure, the patient will show signs of**

   A   dyspnoea, pulmonary oedema and purulent sputum
   B   pulmonary oedema, frothy white sputum and dyspnoea
   C   haemoptysis, generalised oedema and dyspnoea
   D   purulent sputum, generalised oedema and orthopnoea

79. **When an ambulant patient with a history of myocardial infarction complains of chest pain, your first action should be to**

   A   feel for the radial pulse
   B   sit or lie the patient down
   C   record the blood pressure
   D   inform the ward sister

80. **The first cardiac complication of aortic valvular incompetence is**

   A   left atrial hypertrophy
   B   left atrial failure
   C   left ventricular hypertrophy
   D   left ventricular failure

Answers overleaf

76. B 41%

The heart valves close because the pressure of blood in the ventricle is higher than that in the atria. The bicuspid valve is on the left side of the heart and closes when the pressure in the left ventricle is higher than that in the left atrium.

77. A 41%

The soluble plasma protein fibrinogen changes during the clotting process into insoluble fibrin (fibrinogen combines with thrombin to form fibrin).

78. B 73%

Blood normally returns from the lungs to the left atrium then to the left ventricle. However, this process only occurs effectively if the chambers are empty. In ventricular failure, the chambers do not work efficiently, some blood remains in the chamber causing congestion of blood in the pulmonary veins. This, in turn, increases the pressure in the pulmonary capillaries and oedema results, giving rise to poor gas exchange. In addition to dyspnoea, frothy white sputum occurs.

79. B 79%

If a patient complains of chest pains following a myocardial infarction, it indicates that the same pathological process in recurring. The patient should be sat down before the nurse carries out any observations.

80. C 83%

The aortic valve is situated at the opening of the aorta as it leaves the left ventricle. It prevents the back-flow of blood by closing once the ventricle has contracted and pumped blood into aorta. Aortic insufficiency can result from congenital reasons or from rheumatic disease or syphilitic disease.
The result of the incompetence means that blood is allowed to flow back into the left ventricle, which then has to become larger to accommodate the extra blood. The enlargement of the ventricle is known as hypertrophy.

81. The action of the autonomic nervous system helps control

    A   body balance, blushing and gland secretions
    B   running, voice production and body balance
    C   running, voice production and blushing
    D   voice production, body balance and blushing

82. Babinski's sign is

    A   the big toe turning upwards when the sole of the foot is stroked
    B   the big toe turning downwards when the sole of the foot is stroked
    C   flickering of the abdominal muscle when abdomen is stroked
    D   deep tendon ankle jerk

83. The most likely cause of ophthalmia neonatorum in this country is the

    A   streptococcus
    B   staphylococcus
    C   gonococcus
    D   herpes simplex virus

84. Sub-acute degeneration of the spinal cord occurs in

    A   bulbar poliomyelitis
    B   pernicious anaemia
    C   syphilitic gummata
    D   multiple sclerosis

85. A positive Kernig's sign indicates

    A   cerebral haemorrhage
    B   meningitis
    C   neuritis
    D   cerebral tumour

Answers overleaf

81. A 70%

The autonomic nervous system controls the functions of the heart, secreting glands and involuntary muscles, therefore controls body balance, blushing and gland secretions.

82. A 45%

Babinski's sign — the great toe extends upward on stroking the sole of the foot — a sign of an upper motor neurone lesion on the opposite side. Newly born infants normally display a bilateral Babinski response, extended big toe and wide separation of the toes. Within 6 months, this should become a normal plantar response.

83. C 64%

Ophthalmia neonatorum is a gonococcal infection transmitted to an infant from an infected mother during delivery.

84. B 48%

The patient has the usual symptoms of anaemia with a smooth, usually sore tongue and the skin has a lemon-yellow tint. In addition, degeneration of the spinal cord may result in ataxia and occasional paralysis.

85. B 87%

Kernig's sign is the inability to straighten the legs at the knee joint when the thigh is flexed at right angles to the trunk. In meningitis, the meninges are inflamed and, if stretched, intense pain occurs.

86. **Would widely dilated pupils be a characteristic sign of**

    A   hyperventilation
    B   dehydration
    C   pyrexia
    D   extensive brain damage

87. **Which of the following defines a morbid impulse to steal:**

    A   hypomania
    B   kleptomania
    C   pyromania
    D   acute mania

88. **Decreased tendon reflexes are a feature of**

    A   upper motor neurone lesions
    B   lower motor neurone lesions
    C   cerebro-vascular accidents
    D   cerebral tumour

89. **During subarachnoid haemorrhage bleeding occurs**

    A   into the ventricles
    B   between the arachnoid mater and dura mater
    C   between the arachnoid mater and the pia mater
    D   into the frontal lobes

90. **The first sign of cerebral anoxia is**

    A   retrograde amnesia
    B   cyanosis
    C   unconsciousness
    D   restlessness

Answers overleaf

86.　D　89%

Extensive brain damage will affect the third cranial nerve (occulomotor nerve), causing dilated and fixed pupils.

87.　B　92%

Kleptomania is a Greek word meaning:—
klepto — I steal; mania — frenzy.
Therefore, kleptomania means uncontrollable and irrational impulse to steal.

88.　B　46%

The reflex action is a function of the lower motor neurone. If, therefore, a lesion occurs, the reflex action will be decreased or absent.

89.　C　74%

The arachnoid mater is the middle layer of the three meninges which surround and protect the brain. Immediately against the brain is the pia mater, the next layer is the arachnoid mater and the outer third layer which is composed of two layers is the dura mater. A sub-arachnoid haemorrhage occurs between the arachnoid mater and the pia mater. It is in this space that the cerebral spinal fluid circulates, so that any haemorrhage into this space will be demonstrated when a lumbar puncture withdraws cerebral spinal fluid.

90.　D　64%

The first sign of cerebral anoxia is restlessness as the brain cannot function as normal without a rich supply of oxygen. Whilst anoxia may lead to memory change, cyanosis, and unconsciousness, it is restlessness which will occur initially.

91. Increasing intracranial pressure is indicated by

    A   rising blood pressure and a rapid, thready pulse

    B   rising blood pressure and a slowing, full pulse

    C   falling blood pressure and a rapid, thready pulse

    D   falling blood pressure and a slowing, full pulse

92. Upper motor neurone disease produces

    A   spasticity with exageration of reflex

    B   spasticity with loss of reflex

    C   flaccidity with exageration of reflex

    D   flaccidity with loss of reflex

93. Menière's disease results from

    A   degeneration of the semi-circular canals

    B   increased pressure of the endolymph in the inner ear

    C   increased pressure of the endolymph in the middle ear

    D   blockage of the eustachian tubes

94. The senior nurse in charge of an unconscious patient should

    A   maintain silence while attending to the patient

    B   assist the junior nurse with the administration of oral fluids

    C   teach the junior nurse about the patient's condition while carrying out nursing care

    D   ensure the patient's position is changed at least every two hours and more frequently if possible

95. In order to give individualised care to a patient suffering from multiple sclerosis, it will be most useful for the nurse to be aware of the

    A   progressive nature of the illness

    B   drug regime and likely side effects

    C   patient's history and social background

    D   psychological effects of disability

Answers overleaf

91. B   76%

As intracranial pressure increases, a rise in blood pressure and a slowing pulse occurs due to the hypoxic stimulus of the vasomotor centre.

92. A   22%

The upper motor neurones arise from the motor cortex of the cerebrum and run in the descending pyramidal tract to the spinal cord. They produce and modify muscular movement. If a lesion occurs, then increased muscle tone occurs, causing spasticity but the reflexes remain as these are a function of the lower motor neurones.

93. B   39%

Menière's disease results from increased pressure of the endolymph in the inner ear. There is no known cause but there is an increase in the amount of endolymph within the semi-circular canals causing tinnitus (ringing in the ears), vertigo (dizziness), and progressive nerve deafness.

94. D   66%

An unconscious patient is defined as being in a deep abnormal sleep of unknown duration without reflex actions. One of the last senses to go is believed to be hearing, so a nurse should talk to the patient and explain the procedures being carried out in an attempt not only to arouse the patient, but also to allow him to know what is going on. As the patient may be able to hear, it is important not to say anything in the patient's hearing which would be detrimental to their condition or upset them. The patient may not have the reflex actions of swallowing or coughing, therefore the nurse should not administer fluids. The nursing care of an unconscious patient involves assessing their needs, planning the care and implementing the plan. Due to the fact that the patient is not moving, it is important to change the patient's position at least every two hours to prevent the hazards of immobility.

95. C   70%

In order to give individualised care it is important for nursing staff to know the specific problems and capabilities of the patient. Whilst the other options are also important, C is essential.

96. **A patient has a large space-occupying lesion and developed total blindness quite rapidly. The lesion is probably**

   A   intra-ocular
   B   in front of the chiasma
   C   at the chiasma
   D   behind the chiasma

97. **Which of the following signs would occur first if a patient was bleeding after a tonsillectomy:**

   A   pallor
   B   restlessness
   C   increased swallowing
   D   tachycardia

98. **Atropine eye drops are instilled when a patient has a detached retina in order to**

   A   reduce intra-ocular pressure
   B   produce constricted pupils
   C   relieve the pain
   D   produce a good view of the fundus oculi

99. **Nystagmus is best defined as**

   A   lack of co-ordination of the external eye muscles
   B   a fixed deviation of either eye from its's normal direction
   C   rapid, involuntary movement of the eyeball
   D   drooping of the eyelid due to loss of nervous control

100. **An epileptic patient prescribed phenytoin sodium (Epanutin), may as a result develop**

   A   diarrhoea
   B   gum hyperplasia
   C   nephrotic syndrome
   D   tinnitus

Answers overleaf

96.   C   43%

Space-occupying lesions can affect vision because of compression on the visual pathways. Any lesion of the visual pathway results in some degree of blindness. Options A, B and D can produce blindness in one eye (and partial blindness in other eye in case of option D). Only lesions at the chiasma, the crossover of the visual pathway, cause total blindness in both eyes.

97.   C   78%

The tonsils are in the oropharynx and are very vascular. If the tonsillar bed bleeds post-operatively, the patient will swallow the blood.

98.   D   61%

Atropine dilates the pupil — a necessary preparation if an ophthalmoscope is used to examine the nature and extent of the retinal detachment. Pain and raised intraocular pressure are not features of this condition.

99.   C   75%

This may be caused by disease of the semi-circular canals, or the central nervous system. Lack of co-ordination of external eye muscles would lead to diplopia. Strabismus results from a fixed deviation of either eye from its' normal direction. Drooping of the upper lid is termed ptosis.

100.   B   53%

Gum hyperplasia (thickening) is a side effect of phenytoin sodium and should be watched for by nursing staff when patients are prescribed this drug.

101. The cause of unconsciousness in a patient suffering from a hyperglycaemic coma is likely to be

A   dehydration
B   high blood sugar level
C   ketosis
D   electrolyte imbalance

102. Which one of the following is a function of oestrogen:

A   preparation of the ova for fertilisation
B   regeneration of the endometrium
C   development of the placenta for the implanted ova
D   separation of the endometrium at menstruation

103. Patients suffering from Addison's disease require regular doses of

A   adrenocorticotrophic hormone
B   cortisone
C   sodium chloride
D   potassium chloride

104. Acromegaly is likely to occur in

A   a baby
B   an infant
C   an adolescent
D   an adult

105. Diabetes insipidus occurs when there are changes in the

A   pancreas
B   anterior lobe of the pituitary gland
C   adrenal cortex
D   posterior lobe of the pituitary gland

Answers overleaf

101.   C   58%

Ketosis is the first thing one thinks of as the cause of coma in hyperglycaemia, and this must represent the answer. Sugar is not itself a toxin, even in diabetes. However, in the presence of excess blood sugar, fats are incompletely metabolised and ketone bodies are formed; this is ketosis. These ketones are toxic and cause the coma typical of hyperglycaemia. Acetone which appears in the urine is evidence of this ketosis.

102.   B   43%

Preparation of the ovum is under the control of follicle stimulating hormone released by the anterior pituitary gland. Development of the placenta and separation of the endometrium are controlled by progesterone.

103.   B   55%

Addison's disease is due to underactivity of the adrenal gland and a reduced production of cortisol. Cortisone is used therapeutically to replace the cortisol.

104.   D   82%

In an adult, acromegaly is caused by over-production of the human growth hormone from the anterior lobe of the pituitary gland. (See also question 106)

105.   D   30%

The posterior lobe of the pituitary gland produces antidiuretic hormone (ADH). If there is a reduced production of ADH, diabetes insipidus occurs because excessive water is excreted in the urine as a result of a lack of the anti-diuretic hormone.

106. **Acromegaly results from an increased function of the**

    A   pituitary gland
    B   parathyroid gland
    C   adrenal gland
    D   thyroid gland

107. **In thyrotoxicosis, which one of the following may be prescribed:**

    A   Neo-Medrone
    B   Neobacrin
    C   Neo-Mercazole
    D   Neo-Cytamen

108. **Phaeochromocytoma is a tumour known to affect the**

    A   adrenal cortex
    B   adrenal medulla
    C   pituitary gland
    D   thymus gland

109. **Which surgery may be performed in a severe case of myasthenia gravis:**

    A   hypophysectomy
    B   adrenalectomy
    C   parathyroidectomy
    D   thymectomy

110. **Which of the following is a function of insulin:**

    A   converting stored glycogen into glucose
    B   aiding the absorption of glucose in the ileum
    C   facilitating the uptake of glucose by the cell
    D   aiding the digestion of carbohydrate

Answers overleaf

106. A 75%

Acromegaly is marked enlargement of bones, especially of the jaw, hands and feet. It is caused by over-secretion of the growth hormone produced by the over-activity of the anterior lobe of the pituitary gland. In children, over-activity produces excessive growth in size and height — Gigantism. In the adult, the bone does not enlarge but the soft tissue does so that the patient's normal size of rings, shoes and dentures changes. The further effects are amenorrhoea, impotence, diabetes, arthritis and possibly compression on the optic pathways.

107. C 60%

Neo-Mercazole (Carbimazole) is an anti-thyroid drug, reducing the amount of thyroxine produced. It inhibits uptake of iodine by the gland.

108. B 21%

Phaeochromocytoma is a tumour of the adrenal medulla causing high blood levels of adrenaline and noradrenaline. The action of the sympathetic nervous system is potentiated.

109. D 38%

Myasthenia gravis is a disease of the nervous system which affects the junction between the nerves and the muscles. It is thought to be auto-immune based. The eye muscles are usually affected first and there is drooping of the eyelids and double vision. The muscles of chewing and swallowing are also affected, as are respiratory muscles. The treatment involves regulating exertion and drugs. PROSTIGMIN is the drug of choice. Thymectomy, removal of the thymus gland, may result in remission of symptoms because of the gland processes antibody producing cells.

110. C 60%

Insulin facilitates the uptake of glucose by the cell. It's primary role is to regulate the rate of glucose transfer across the cell membranes. The rate of glucose utilisation in the tissue cells is directly related to the amount of insulin present.

111. **A patient develops a thyroid crisis. The immediate nursing action would be**

A   to give plenty of water to drink
B   to reduce the pyrexia and administer sedation as prescribed by the doctor
C   to give plenty of glucose fluids to drink
D   to send the patient back to the operating department for wound exploration

112. **The hormone secreted by the parathyroid glands controls the**

A   amount of sodium excreted
B   metabolic rate
C   level of calcium in the blood
D   state of mental alertness

113. **The anti-diuretic hormone is produced by the**

A   hypothalmus
B   anterior lobe of the pituitary gland
C   posterior lobe of the pituitary gland
D   adrenal glands

114. **In tetany there will be a low blood level of**

A   chlorides
B   potassium
C   sodium
D   calcium

115. **Which one of the following is *most* likely to be observed at the onset of a hyperglycaemic coma:**

A   moist pale skin
B   weak and irregular pulse
C   dry inelastic skin
D   abdominal pain

Answers overleaf

111. B 80%

A thyroid crisis is an acute episode producing all the symptoms of thyrotoxicosis. The major features include restlessness, delirium, tachycardia, hyperpyrexia and vasomotor collapse. The crisis may be precipitated by infections, unusual emotional stress or labour but most often by surgery. Treatment is urgent.

112. C 83%

Parathormone is secreted by the parathyroid glands and controls the plasma calcium concentration.

113. C 42%

The anti-diuretic hormone is produced by the posterior lobe of the pituitary gland. This hormone regulates diuresis by governing the amount of water reabsorbed by the distal and collecting tubules of the kidney.

114. D 81%

Tetany is an increased excitability of the nerves due to a reduced serum calcium level. Carpo-pedal spasm is an early sign of the muscle spasms which result.

115. C 38%

A dry inelastic skin is a very common feature at the onset of hyperglycaemic coma. This is evidence of the dehydration resulting from the diuresis preceding coma. Occasionally, abdominal pain may herald coma too, but this is not as common as a dry inelastic skin.

116. **A patient suffering from severe uncontrolled diabetes mellitus typically has a**

    A   lowered blood glucose level
    B   raised urinary specific gravity
    C   raised blood volume
    D   raised arterial pressure of carbon dioxide (pCO_2)

117. **Immediately following a partial thyroidectomy, a doctor should be summoned if the nurse observes**

    A   a slow pulse
    B   a high temperature
    C   pallor
    D   cessation of drainage

118. **Progesterone levels fall**

    A   if the ovum is fertilised
    B   after rupture of the ovarian folicle
    C   after degeneration of the corpus luteum
    D   after ovulation

119. **A patient with untreated diabetes loses weight and tires easily because**

    A   he drinks too much and eats too little
    B   his diet is high in carbohydrates
    C   he has frequency of micturition
    D   he is unable to metabolise blood sugar

120. **Following an insulin injection, a diabetic patient complains of blurred vision and a cold, clammy skin. The nurse should *first* of all**

    A   prepare dextrose for injection
    B   give the patient 50 gm glucose in water
    C   test the patient's urine for sugar and ketones
    D   check the type and amount of insulin given

Answers overleaf

116. **B   64%**

In diabetes mellitus, the blood sugar level is higher than the so called "renal threshold" and sugar is excreted in the urine. Commonly, the urine is pale and with a specific gravity of 1026 or more.

117. **B   29%**

During removal of part of the thyroid gland, thyroxine may be released in a high concentration into the blood stream. This will increase the metabolic rate causing a rise in temperature and may indicate onset of a thyroid crisis.

118. **C   65%**

The corpus luteum produces progesterone; therefore, when the corpus luteum degenerates, the progesterone level will fall.

119. **D   83%**

Insulin allows metabolism of glucose and energy production. If glucose cannot be utilised, the patient feels tired and as fat and protein is used instead, the patient loses weight.

120. **B   54%**

Insulin allows glucose to be metabolised; however, if hypoglycaemia results, the patient will feel unwell and complain of blurred vision and a cold, clammy skin. Glucose needs to be given quickly.

121. **Which of the following gives a patient a painless movable joint:**

A   arthrodesis
B   arthroplasty
C   arthroscopy
D   arthrosis

122. **The first stage in the healing of fractures is**

A   callus formation
B   osteoblast activity
C   haematoma formation
D   deposition of mineral salts

123. **A rotational force may cause a fracture of which type:**

A   oblique
B   compound
C   comminuted
D   spiral

124. **A patient with rheumatic fever is ordered prolonged bed rest to**

A   protect and immobilise his painful, swollen joints
B   limit accumulation of tissue fluid
C   limit the possibility of heart damage
D   prevent joint deformities

125. **Internal fixation means that**

A   the joint of the bone is immobilised in a fixed position
B   an anaesthetic was necessary to reduce the fracture
C   the broken bone has been permanently attached to a stronger
    bone
D   a support such as a Thomas Splint has been applied to
    stabilise the bone

Answers overleaf

121. B 68%

Arthroplasty means reconstruction of a joint giving a painless
movable joint. Arthrodesis is fixation of a movable joint;
arthroscopy is examination of a joint and arthrosis refers to
articulation.

122. C 85%

A haematoma is formed when a fracture occurs and initiates the
healing process.

123. D 47%

A fracture is a break in the continuity of a bone, usually caused
by an injury. The injury may be from direct or indirect violence or
from muscle action. Some fractures are defined depending on the
direction of the fracture, i.e. Spiral — winding continually.

124. C 58%

Rheumatic endocarditis is a significant complication of this
condition. Mitral stenosis and embolic diseases are serious
sequelae of this complication. Protection and immobilisation of
involved joints is a secondary consideration only.

125. B 57%

Internal fixation or splinting is carried out by an open operation
which fixes the fractured ends of the bone by the insertion of
screws, plates and intramedullary nails. The advantages of internal
splinting are:
  (i)   the fracture is held in accurate reduction and so healing is
        encouraged;
  (ii) it makes it easier to nurse the patient and enables the
        patient to move around the bed;
  (iii) the patient can exercise his limb independently;
  (iv) internal fixation can allow earlier weight-bearing.

126. **A Smith-Peterson pin is used to treat a fractured**

A shaft of femur
B tibia
C humerus
D neck of femur

127. **Which of the following statements best describes the usual pattern of joint involvement in rheumatic fever:**

A only large joints are affected
B symptoms tend to move from joint to joint
C small joints are never affected
D joint deformities are common once the acute attack is over

128. **Which of the following best describes the term "fracture reduction":**

A making the bone smaller by removing the bone fragments
B manual manipulation of the broken bone and surrounding muscles
C surgical removal of bone tissues
D bringing the two ends of the bone into proper alignment

129. **Which one of the following is the immediate nursing priority following a total hip replacement:**

A turning patient onto the unaffected side to relieve pressure
B prevention of deep vein thrombosis with passive exercises
C avoiding constipation with a high fibre diet
D prevention of dislocation of the hip

130. **A seven year old child has a supracondylar fracture. The *most* important observation to make is of her**

A pulse and blood pressure
B wrist and finger movements
C blood pressure and temperature
D pulse at the affected wrist

Answers overleaf

126. D   39%

A Smith-Peterson pin is one way of using internal fixation to treat a fractured neck of femur. The pin or nail is used to treat fractures of the neck of the femur if the fracture can be reduced accurately and if the patient is young. In older patients, or when reduction would not provide accurate union, an Austin-Moore prosthesis or Thompson's prosthesis is used. These prostheses allow the patient to mobilise earlier and therefore prevent problems of bed rest. Fractures of the shaft of the femur require skeletal traction with a Thomas's splint or an operation using a Küntscher nail as internal fixation. Fracture of the tibia requires manipulation to allow the bone ends to heal in position and then either a plaster of paris to hold bones in alignment or an open reduction with the introduction of an intra-medullary nail. Fractures of the humerus, as with all fractures, have the bone ends aligned and are then held in position with a plaster of paris.

127. B   59%

Rheumatic fever is a disease affecting many parts of the body but particularly the joints. The patient complains of migratory joint pains.

128. D   77%

In fracture reduction, the two ends of bone are brought into alignment to allow the healing process to take place to maintain conformity of the bone.

129. D   80%

The patient must be positioned carefully with the affected leg in abduction and the hip flexed less than 45° to prevent dislocation.

130. D   57%

The supracondylar fracture occurs at the lower end of the humerus. If the fracture becomes displaced, it may affect the brachial artery or the nerve, so it is important to assess the radial pulse on the injured arm to be alert for any artery damage.

131. Phimosis is

   A   constriction of the prepuce so that it cannot be retracted

   B   a malformation in which the urethra opens on the under surface of the penis

   C   a malformation in which the urethra lies open anteriorly along the shaft of the penis

   D   absence of the kidneys leading to hydronephrosis

132. The temperature of the average normal female during child-bearing age is

   A   the same throughout the monthly cycle

   B   higher the first half of the cycle, lower from ovulation to the next cycle

   C   lower for the first half of the cycle, higher from ovulation to the next cycle

   D   lower at the beginning of the cycle, rises at ovulation, lowers a few days after this

133. A nullipara is

   A   a woman who is pregnant for the first time

   B   the name given to a woman at the end of her first labour and thereafter

   C   a woman who has not had any children

   D   a woman who has had more than one child

134. Hydramnios is

   A   insufficient amount of amniotic fluid

   B   excessive fluid in the ventricles of the brain

   C   insufficient fluid in the ventricles of the brain

   D   excessive amount of amniotic fluid

135. Menorrhagia means

   A   normal blood loss at the time of the menstrual period

   B   excessive blood loss at the time of the menstrual period

   C   diminished blood loss at the time of the menstrual period

   D   excessive blood loss between the normal menstrual period

Answers overleaf

131.   **A**   **74%**

Phimosis is the constriction of the prepuce so that it cannot be retracted over the glans penis, causing oedema and pain.

132.   **D**   **90%**

The temperature during the menstrual cycle rises slightly during ovulation. It is due to the corpus luteum producing progesterone.

133.   **C**   **79%**

A nullipara is a woman who has never given birth to a child. Multipara is a woman who has had more than one pregnancy. Unipara is a woman who has had only one child. Primigravida is a woman who is pregnant for the first time.

134.   **D**   **82%**

Hydramnios is an excessive amount of amniotic fluid — the watery fluid in which the foetus floats in the uterus until birth. It occurs more often in the diabetic patient. It is uncomfortable for the patient and causes foetal complications. Amniocentesis is the taking of amniotic fluid — it can indicate whether there are any gross abnormalities in the foetus.

135.   **B**   **81%**

Menorrhagia means prolonged and increased blood loss during a regular period. Fibroids are a common cause, and if menorrhagia remains untreated, anaemia will develop.

136. **Which operation corrects an anterior vaginal wall prolapse:**

A   colpoperineorrhaphy
B   oophorectomy
C   colporrhaphy
D   ventro-suspension

137. **Hutchinson's teeth may be seen in a patient suffering from**

A   gonorrhoea
B   congenital syphilis
C   tetracycline overdose
D   trichomonas vaginalis

138. **A positive pregnancy test performed on urine depends on the presence of**

A   progesterone
B   17 ketosteroids
C   chorionic gonadotrophin
D   5 hydroxytryptomine

139. **The *most* important aspect of antenatal care in helping to produce a healthy mother and baby is**

A   gaining co-operation of mother-to-be
B   urine testing and recording of blood pressure
C   taking blood for examination
D   taking a full history

140. **Checking for residual urine entails**

A   calculating urinary output prior to catheterisation
B   catheterisation of the patient at 6am and 6pm
C   releasing a catheter clamp 4 hourly
D   catheterisation of the patient after micturition

Answers overleaf

136.   C   54%

Colpoperineorrhaphy is the repair of a torn vagina and perineum. Oophorectomy means removal of an ovary. Ventro-suspension is an operation to suture abdominal viscera to the anterior abdominal wall.

137.   B   58%

Congenital syphilis is becoming rare as a routine Wasserman test carried out on women at antenatal clinics can demonstrate the disease. The disease can then be treated. Congenital syphilis shows the following signs: failure to gain weight, under-developed nasal bones causing depressed bridge of the nose, and a scaly, yellow or copper-coloured rash. Later in childhood, notches appear in incisor teeth of the second dentition — these are known as Hutchinson's Teeth. Tetracycline overdose shows with yellow discolouration of teeth and inhibition of bone growth in children.

138.   C   64%

Chorionic gonadotrophin is secreted into the fluids of the mother by the cells of the fertilised ovum. The secretion of this hormone can first be measured after ovulation, just as the ovum is first implanting in the endometrium. The rate of excretion rises rapidly to reach a maximum approximately seven weeks after ovulation and decreases to a relatively low value by 16 weeks after ovulation.

139.   D   47%

It must be ensured that the pregnant woman has no condition that will affect her or the foetus during pregnancy — a full medical history must be taken.

140.   D   84%

The aim is to check how well the bladder is emptying, hence the need for catheterisation to be performed immediately after the patient has passed urine.

141. **Which tests may be used to confirm the diagnosis of infectious mononucleosis:**

A   Paul Bunnell and Trousseau
B   Wassermann and Kahn
C   Paul Bunnell and Monospot
D   Schick and Queckensted

142. **Reverse barrier nursing would be carried out on a patient suffering from**

A   infective hepatitis
B   tuberculosis
C   leukaemia
D   scabies

143. **A toxoid is a**

A   toxin deprived of some of its harmful properties
B   suspension of killed organisms in normal saline
C   suspension of killed organisms
D   toxin not deprived of harmful properties

144. **Koplik's spots appear in**

A   measles
B   rubella
C   scarlet fever
D   chicken pox

145. **Immunisation with triple vaccine is usually begun by the age of**

A   1 month
B   3 months
C   6 months
D   9 months

Answers overleaf

141.   C   21%

Mononucleosis (Glandular fever) is caused by a virus and can be diagnosed by using the Paul Bunnell and Monospot tests. WR and Kahn confirm syphillis; Schick test aids in the diagnosis of diptheria and Queckensted's test entails compression of the jugular vein during lumbar puncture.

142.   C   87%

Reverse barrier nursing is used to protect the patient from infection and used for the leukaemic patient as they are prone to infection due to the low number of mature white blood cells.

143.   A   64%

Many toxins are too dangerous to administer to human beings. They are modified so that they are harmless yet confer immunity, for example diptheria toxoid is a toxin which has been treated with formaldehyde.

144.   A   57%

In measles, Koplik's spots occur on the mucous membrane of the cheeks. They are tiny white spots present during the prodromal stage, before onset of other symptoms.

145.   B   69%

The Department of Health and Social Security recommended that triple vaccine is commenced at the age of 3 months.

146.   Natural passive immunity results from

    A   contracting the disease and recovering
    B   placental transfer
    C   a subclinical attack
    D   vaccination

147.   The pathogen responsible for gas gangrene is

    A   staphylococcus aureus
    B   haemolytic streptococcus
    C   staphylococcus albus
    D   clostridium welchii

148.   An injection of gamma globulin provides

    A   natural acquired active immunity
    B   natural acquired passive immunity
    C   artificial acquired active immunity
    D   artificial acquired passive immunity

149.   Which of the following is the reason for pain experienced with inflammatory response:

    A   pressure on the nerve endings due to oedema
    B   extra heat in the area
    C   bacterial activity on the pain fibres
    D   plasma proteins in the tissue space

150.   Severe anaphylaxis is caused by

    A   sudden release of adrenaline
    B   hypersensitivity to foreign protein
    C   sudden severe bronchospasm
    D   hypersensitivity to histamine

Answers overleaf

146. B 75%

Natural passive immunity is passed from mother to baby. By immunity is meant the ability of an individual to resist disease. All passive immunity is short-lived. A newborn baby is passively immunised to diseases to which his mother is immune.

147. D 85%

Clostridium welchii causes gas gangrene. This serious and often fatal disease is caused by this anaerobic organism. Extensive contaminated wounds permit entry of the organism, which can thrive in the absence of oxygen. Stored glucogen in the muscles is the food supply and a noxious and evil-smelling gas is liberated in the wound, hence the name gas gangrene.

148. D 30%

Gamma globulin contains specific antibodies made by a human donor. It thus confers passive immunity when injected into a human recipient. It is artificially acquired as the recipient does not make it himself.

149. A 79%

Pressure on the nerve endings due to oedema is the reason for pain experienced with the inflammatory response. The pressure irritates the nerve endings and is interpreted by the brain as a painful stimuli.

150. B 69%

Often referred to as anaphylactic shock, it is a severe allergic response to a foreign protein. Urgent treatment is essential to counteract this potentially fatal condition. Adrenaline, hydrocortisone and antihistamine therapy may be prescribed.

151. **Which one of the following is a contagious skin disease:**

    A   impetigo
    B   herpes simplex
    C   eczema
    D   contact dermatitis

152. **A characteristic of a malignant tumour is**

    A   the growth is contained within a capsule
    B   the initial tumour can infiltrate into surrounding tissue
    C   the rate of development is slow
    D   the cell structure is identical to that of the parent cell

153. **"Erythema" is**

    A   slight bruising
    B   superficial redness
    C   local swelling
    D   marked itching

154. **A skin condition which is a sympton of advanced cirrhosis of the liver is**

    A   sycosis barbae
    B   erythema nodosum
    C   rosacea
    D   spider naevi

155. **Herpes zoster is closely associated with**

    A   bronchopneumonia
    B   chicken pox
    C   urticaria
    D   pemphigus

Answers overleaf

151.   A   88%

Impetigo is an acute contagious inflammation of the skin of streptococcal or staphylococcal origin. Pustules and scabs are present on the skin.

152.   B   91%

The characteristic of a malignant tumour is that the initial tumour can infiltrate into surrounding tissue. Tumours are called malignant when they grow rapidly, tend to infiltrate surrounding healthy tissues, and to spread to distant parts of the body, leading eventually to death.

153.   B   75%

Erythema is superficial reddening of the skin.

154.   D   45%

Skin conditions which are symptoms of advanced cirrhosis of the liver are spider naevi. These are small red areas surrounded by a dilated capillary network which resembles a spider's web, found on the skin of the abdomen and thorax.

155.   B   85%

The virus herpes zoster is closely related to the chicken pox virus. In some cases of shingles it can be shown that there has been contact with a person suffering from chicken pox.

156. A 30 year old lady is admitted to the ward with fever, localised eruption on the front of the legs, raised indurated red tender nodes. These features could describe

  A   urticaria
  B   erythema multiforme
  C   erythema nodosum
  D   alopecia areata

157. In the skin, the epidermal cells are continually being manufactured by the

  A   stratum spinosum
  B   stratum lucidum
  C   stratum germinativum
  D   stratum corneum

158. Ringworm is caused by a:

  A   fungus
  B   worm
  C   insect
  D   virus

159. Which of the following would best indicate how much fluid is needed in the early stages of a severe burn:

  A   blood pressure
  B   level of consciousness
  C   percentage of body surface burned
  D   urine output

160. The most effective method of lowering the temperature of a pyrexial patient is to

  A   dry the skin thoroughly at frequent intervals
  B   provide air movement to assist with evaporation of sweat
  C   keep the patient warm to enhance sweating
  D   give ice to suck and copious iced fluids

Answers overleaf

156. C 42%

Erythema nodosum is an inflammatory disease of the skin and subcutaneous tissue characterised by tender red nodules more commonly found below the knees and on the forearms. It is most common in young adults. The nodules change colour from pink to bluish-brown, resembling a bruise. Urticaria is an allergic skin reaction to drugs, insect stings or bites, injections or certain foods. The reaction causes local wheals and erythema, a superficial redness of the skin. Erythema multiforme is an acute eruption of the skin which may be due to an allergy or drug sensitivity. It occurs primarily on the hands, feet and mucous membrane. Alopecia areata — sudden loss of hair with no obvious skin disorder. The scalp and beard are most commonly involved.

157. C 79%

The stratum germinativum produces new epidermal cells.

158. A 55%

Ringworm is caused by fungi which usually infect the hair causing bald red patches to occur.

159. C 76%

The amount of fluid lost in burns is calculated by the percentage of body surface burned and the patient's weight.

160. B 73%

The cooling process is enhanced if sweat on the skin is allowed to dry naturally, rather than be dried deliberately with a towel. Air movement will therefore aid the evaporation of sweat and help cool the patient.

DRUGS AND THERAPEUTIC HAZARDS

161.   A solution of normal saline is

    A   isotonic
    B   hypotonic
    C   catatonic
    D   hypertonic

162.   In which of the following drug classifications would sodium cromoglycate (Intal) be included:

    A   bronchodilator
    B   antibiotic
    C   antihistamine
    D   tranquilliser

163.   The organs of the body most susceptible to damage from ionising radiations are the

    A   adrenals
    B   thyroid/parathyroids
    C   gonads
    D   lungs

164.   An elderly patient refuses to swallow his drugs. Should you

    A   leave him alone and try again later
    B   make a note of his refusal and report it
    C   firmly but politely insist he swallows them
    D   ask medical staff to prescribe the drug for intramuscular administration

165.   Atropine will

    A   increase the resting heart rate
    B   weaken skeletal muscle
    C   increase flow of saliva
    D   increase activity of the small intestine

Answers overleaf

161.   A   65%

Isotonic means "equal tension". Normal saline (0.9% solution of salt in water) is a physiological fluid and has the same osmotic pressure as blood.

162.   C   54%

Sodium cromoglycate (Intal) is an antihistamine used in prevention rather than treatment. It is thought to interfere with the release of histamine during an antigen/antibody reaction, helping to prevent oedema and narrowing of the respiratory tract.

163.   C   66%

The gonads contain rapidly dividing cells that carry genetic material and are prone to damage by ionising radiation. If they are damaged by radiation, sterility can occur. It must, therefore, be ensured that they receive the minimum dosage of radiation per year.

164.   B   66%

Making a note of the patient's refusal to swallow his drugs and reporting the incident to sister is the wisest course of action. Insisting that the patient complies with your wishes will only heighten the patient's anxiety and may provoke an unpleasant situation. Prescribing intramuscular administration is pointless; the patient is at liberty to refuse that too.

165.   A   60%

Atropine inhibits the effect of the vagus nerve on the heart causing tachycardia. It also inhibits respiratory and gastric secretions, dilates the pupils and relaxes muscle spasm.

166. Hydroxocobalamin (Neo-Cytamen) is given

A in tablet form
B initially by intravenous infusion
C by intramuscular injection
D by subcutaneous injection

167. Adrenaline has the effect of converting

A glycogen to glucose
B glucose to glycogen
C glycogen to glucagon
D glucagon to glycogen

168. The most dangerous side-effect of prolonged administration of cortisone is

A the appearance of sugar in the urine
B masked infection
C development of moon face
D retention of body fluid

169. The Paediatric stock of Digoxin contains 0.05 mg per ml. A child to have 0.035 mg of Digoxin would require

A 0.7 ml
B 1.2 ml
C 0.4 ml
D 0.1 ml

170. Which drug may have an effect on the neuromuscular junction:

A papaveretum
B diazepam
C suxamethonium
D pentobarbitone

Answers overleaf

166.   C   67%

Hydroxocobalamin (Vitamin B12) is used to treat pernicious anaemia. It is given by intramuscular injection because if given orally, the drug would not be absorbed. An alternative drug given by intramuscular injection in order to treat pernicious anaemia is cyanocobalamin (Cytamen).

167.   A   64%

Adrenaline from the adrenal medulla aids in the conversion of stored glycogen back to glucose, ready for utilisation by the body cells.

168.   B   59%

Although each alternative is a side effect of steroid administration, the *most* dangerous is the masked or delayed signs of any developing infection. For example, a patient with appendicitis receiving steroid therapy may not complain of any signs or symptoms until perforation of the appendix occurs, with resulting peritonitis.

169.   A   90%

Divide the quantity you want by the quantity you have:—

$$\frac{0.035 \text{ mg}}{0.05 \text{ mg}} \times \frac{1}{1} \quad OR \quad \frac{35}{50} \times \frac{1}{1} = \frac{7}{10} \quad OR \quad 0.7 \text{ ml}$$

170.   C   34%

Where a motor nerve meets a muscle, i.e. the 'neuromuscular junction', a small gap occurs. For the nervous impulse to be able to bridge the gap, a chemical transmitter is released, i.e. Acetylcholine. Suxamethonium blocks the neuromuscular transmission.

171. **A patient receiving streptomycin injections would have the treatment discontinued if**

    A   there was abscess formation in the injection site
    B   he complained of ringing in the ears
    C   his temperature was elevated
    D   there was little improvement in the condition

172. **The antidote to warfarin is**

    A   vitamin K
    B   protamine sulphate
    C   streptokinase
    D   phenindione

173. **Administration of suxamethonium (Scoline) leads to**

    A   reduced secretions
    B   return of cough reflex
    C   muscular relaxation
    D   euphoric states

174. **The most common side effect of indomethacin is**

    A   vertigo
    B   gastritis
    C   skin rashes
    D   hypotension

175. **After the administration of insulin, it**

    A   is activated by pancreozymin
    B   delays glycogen storage
    C   enhances glucose utilisation
    D   is destroyed by trypsinogen

Answers overleaf

171.   **B**   76%

Ringing in the ears (tinnitus) is a side-effect of streptomycin injections. It can damage the eighth cranial nerve; other side effects are vertigo, headache and deafness, all related to eighth nerve damage.

172.   **A**   69%

Warfarin is an anti-coagulant which interferes with the formation of the clotting factor by the liver. Overdosages produce haemorrhages which are controlled by vitamin K. Heparin is an anti-coagulant, protamine sulphate is the antidote of this. Streptokinase is used in thrombotic or embolic disease. There is no specific antidote to streptokinase, a blood transfusion would be given in the case of haemorrhage. Phenindione is an anti-coagulant with an action similar to warfarin.

173.   **C**   55%

Suxamethonium rapidly produces profound muscular relaxation of brief duration (less than 5 minutes). It facilitates endotracheal intubation and is also useful in electroconvulsive therapy (ECT). Normal individuals possess an enzyme (cholinesterase) which destroys suxamethonium, but some individuals exist who cannot destroy the drug. These patients fail to resume spontaneous breathing after suxamethonium administration and have to be maintained on a mechanical ventilator until the relaxant has been excreted.

174.   **B**   53%

Indomethacin is a potent drug that can cause serious side effects and toxic effects. It may cause peptic ulceration and gastric irritation and is contra-indicated in patients who have peptic ulcer, gastritis or ulcerative colitis.

175.   **C**   86%

Insulin has its principle use in the control of symptoms of diabetes mellitus when this disease cannot satisfactorily be controlled by diet alone. Insulin is given subcutaneously into the loose connective tissues of the body, usually into the arms or thighs. It cannot be given by mouth because it is destroyed by digestive enzymes.

176. Cortisone is given with milk to

    A decrease peptic ulceration
    B decrease vomiting
    C aid absorption
    D increase the pH of the stomach

177. Which one of the following should be reported immediately if you are caring for a patient having a blood transfusion:

    A headache
    B tingling in the fingers
    C muscular cramp
    D pain in the loins

178. The most important single factor in the treatment of a teenager suffering from drug dependency is to

    A establish a therapeutic relationship
    B prevent his access to drugs
    C initiate aversion therapy
    D admit him to a drug unit

179. Which of the following actions is the *most* dangerous:

    A injecting potassium directly into the intravenous infusion tubing
    B injecting potassium into an intravenous infusion fluid
    C commencing isotonic saline instead of saline 0.9%
    D letting the intravenous infusion run too rapidly

180. Benzyl benzoate is effective against

    A athlete's foot
    B scabies
    C psoriasis
    D pemphigus

Answers overleaf

176. A   51%

Cortisone is an adrenal (glucocorticoid) steroid hormone. It has an anti-inflammatory action and affects fat, protein and carbohydrate metabolism. One of the side effects is gastric ulceration so it is given with milk to coat the gastric lining. Other side effects include retention of salt and water, osteoporosis, muscle wasting, hypertension, diabetes mellitus, weight gain, moon face and cataracts.

177. D   83%

Pain in the loins would indicate that agglutinated red cells were beginning to block the arterioles of the kidney. Oliguria may develop as may haematuria, caused by release of haemoglobin from the agglutinated red cells.

178. A   62%

Without the establishment of a therapeutic relationship, the other three factors proposed would probably have little long-term benefit for the patient.

179. A   64%

Normal rhythmic heart contractions are largely dependent on the correct concentration of potassium, sodium and calcium in the extra cellular fluid. Any change in intravenous administration in rate or solution will alter this. However, the most dangerous is the intravenous injection of potassium into the infusion tubing. If potassium levels are increased in the extra cellular fluid, there is an impairment in conduction and contraction of heart muscle. This causes slowing of the heart and dilatation of the chambers. The pulse becomes slow and cardiac failure can result.

180. B   63%

The itch mite causing scabies is destroyed by application of benzyl benzoate. It is an emulsion applied to the whole of the body after a hot bath, except the head and neck.

STATE FINAL EXAMINATION TECHNIQUE

1. POINTS TO REMEMBER

Objective test examinations are intended to cover a large part of the syllabus, and it is unlikely that you will be able to answer all of the 60 questions easily. It is therefore wise to be prepared for the fact that there may be a small number of questions that you are unable to answer and you should not allow this to spoil your concentration during the examination.

Read the instructions *carefully* before you begin.

The time allocation of 1¼ hours for a 60 item examination may seem generous, but it is intended as 'thinking' time, enabling you to choose the correct answer after careful, reasoned thought. There is only *one* correct answer to each question, but if there seems to you to be more than one possible answer, then read the stem of the question again. There will be some information there to guide you. For example, "Which one of the following is the *most* important" indicates that all four alternatives could be important but one has priority over the rest. Similarly, "Which one of the following must be reported immediately" suggests that all four alternatives may be significant and ought to be reported, but that one deserves *immediate* action.

Note that it is possible to alter your choice of answer *but* you cannot then revert to your original choice, so think carefully before making your decision.

2. MARKING THE COMPUTER SHEET

Only a Grade B (soft) pencil must be used.

Enter your candidate number like this:-

CANDIDATE NUMBER	**0**	**2**	**7**	**1**		0	0	0	0

Write your CANDIDATE NUMBER in the boxes provided AND mark the same figure in the column below each box
Mark the number thus: 4_

0	0	0	0
1	1	1	1
2	2	2	2
3	3	3	3
4	4	4	4
5	5	5	5
6	6	6	6
7	7	7	7
8	8	8	8
9	9	9	9

When answering a question, mark the letter corresponding to the answer you consider correct. There is only one correct answer.

e.g. If you consider the answer to question 1 to be a) mark thus: using heavy pencil lines.

To cancel an answer fill in the bottom of the square thus: and re-mark the correct letter.

Do not use a rubber. It is not possible in the case of question 4 to return to   a) and re-mark it.

	a	b	c	d
1				
2	a	b	c	d
3	a	b	c	d
4		b	c	
5	a	b	c	d
6	a	b	c	d
7	a	b	c	d
8	a	b	c	d
9	a	b	c	d
10	a	b	c	d
11	a	b	c	d
12	a	b	c	d
13	a	b	c	d

You should attempt all 60 questions as marks are not deducted for incorrect answers.

PRACTICE EXAM INSTRUCTIONS

This practice examination has been compiled, as far as possible, to correspond with the range of topics and degree of difficulty which one could expect to find in the SRN Final Examination. Having completed the preceding 180 questions, you will be familiar with the range of topics, but the degree of difficulty of the practice examination questions falls within the range 29%-80%. The very difficult and very easy questions have been omitted in order to provide a realistic examination.

There are 60 questions and the time allowed is 1¼ hours. Do not spend more than the allotted time.

Try to work under conditions which resemble those of the final examination. Do not refer to books, notes or speak to other persons.
Do not smoke — no smoking is allowed during the final examination.

Choose a time when you will be free from distractions and undisturbed, in a well-lit location. A watch or clock should be easily visible.

Answers, with explanations and degree of difficulty (facility value as a %) are to be found on page 91. The pass mark is 50%, i.e. 30 or more correct.

PRACTICE EXAMINATION

60 questions: time allowed 1 ¼ hours

Put a tick against the one answer that you consider to be correct.

1. **The functions of the General Nursing Council are to**

    A   control the training of nurses and midwives
    B   maintain nursing standards in all hospitals in England and
         Wales
    C   prescribe training standards and maintain a register and roll
         of nurses
    D   provide an advisory and legal service relevant to nursing
         practice

2. **The nursing implications of the research entitled "Food for
    Thought" relate to**

    A   nasogastric feeding regimes
    B   pre-operative fasting
    C   effective weight loss programmes
    D   meal choices on hospital menus

3. **You receive a telephone enquiry asking for information about a
    patient's condition. You should**

    A   read the nursing notes and give a summary
    B   consult with the nurse in charge before replying
    C   confirm the enquirers identity then give the information.
    D   explain that the patient is "as well as can be expected"

4. **A baby normally walks holding on to furniture by the age of**

    A   8 months
    B   10 months
    C   13 months
    D   18 months

5. **Swelling occurs following injury because**

A   local sodium levels are increased
B   permeability of capillaries is increased
C   extra cells are present in the area
D   lymphatic drainage is impaired

6. **The majority of newly admitted adult patients are *most* likely to appear**

A   silent, introverted
B   anxious, demanding
C   difficult, agitated
D   confident, calm

7. **A nurse learns that she has just failed her final SRN examination. She comes on duty in an emotional state and is very tearful. The nurse in charge should**

A   send her off duty as she is in no state to nurse sick patients
B   offer her regrets then send the nurse back to work as keeping busy will keep her mind off it
C   try to arrange an urgent counselling session with the clinical teacher and the nurse
D   phone for the nurse's parents or husband to come and console her

8. **One of the first main complications of longstanding chronic bronchitis is**

A   right ventricular failure
B   myocardial ischaemia
C   left ventricular failure
D   angina pectoris

9. **Carbon monoxide poisoning is recognised by**

    A   central cyanosis
    B   intermittent apnoea
    C   pupillary contraction
    D   cherry red skin colouration

10. **When communicating with a deaf patient it is best to**

    A   write most words down in order to avoid confusion
    B   face the patient and speak slowly and clearly
    C   raise your voice whilst standing to one side of the patient
    D   use pictures, symbols and a pointer to avoid misunderstanding

11. **The reason for administering low percentage oxygen to a patient with an acute exacerbation of chronic bronchitis is in order to**

    A   maintain levels of plasma carbon dioxide
    B   reduce levels of oxyhaemoglobin in the blood
    C   maintain respiratory function by anoxic response
    D   prevent the production of carbon dioxide in the tissues

12. **Which is the *most* important aspect of care for a patient with bronchiectasis:**

    A   oxygen therapy
    B   physiotherapy
    C   bronchodilator drugs
    D   antibiotic therapy

13. **Which one of the following is thought to be the cause of coeliac disease:**

    A   an allergic reaction
    B   an infective disorder
    C   a malignant process
    D   a hereditary trait

14. **Removal of the terminal ileum can result in**

    A   iron deficiency anaemia
    B   pernicious anaemia
    C   dumping syndrome
    D   reduced prothrombin levels

15. **Oesophageal varices will occur as a result of raised pressure in the**

    A   portal vein
    B   coeliac artery
    C   hepatic artery
    D   hepatic vein

16. **Jaundice would arise from**

    A   obstruction of the cystic duct
    B   stones in the gall bladder
    C   obstruction of the right hepatic duct
    D   impacted stone at the sphincter of Oddi

17. **A very elderly man in your ward is dying of carcinoma of the liver. He asks if he can have a bottle of beer. You should**

    A give him the beer and say nothing to the rest of the staff
    B give the beer and explain why you did so to the staff
    C gently explain that you can only give alcohol-free drinks to him and suggest ovaltine instead
    D explain that beer is inadvisable since his liver may not be able to detoxicate the alcohol

18. **Following surgery to repair an umbilical hernia, an elderly lady develops retention of urine. *Initially* she requires**

    A diuretics
    B time and privacy
    C extra fluids
    D fluid restriction

19. **The use of peritoneal dialysis is based upon the principle that**

    A the peritoneum allows transfer of substance only from the interior of a vessel outward
    B electrolytes move across a semi-permeable membrane from a higher to a lower concentration
    C when the blood pressure is raised, fluid passes more readily from the blood into the tissues
    D accumulation of toxic metabolities in uraemia render tissue capillaries unusually porus

20. **A high protein diet may be given to a patient with nephrotic syndrome because protein**

    A absorption is delayed in the intestine
    B is required to replace damaged kidney cells
    C is continually passed in the urine
    D is lost from the intestinal wall.

21. **Substances with a high renal threshold**

A   never appear in urine
B   never appear in the filtrate
C   are excreted if the plasma level is too low
D   are excreted if the plasma level is too high

22. **A child on the paediatric ward has threadworms. The *most* important treatment before putting him to bed is to**

A   cut his finger nails
B   give him a bath
C   ensure he has clean pyjamas
D   ensure he has his bowels open

23. **Central venous pressure is an indication of**

A   pressure in the right atrium
B   diastolic blood pressure
C   pressure in the ante cubital vein
D   left ventricular pressure

24. **In left ventricular failure, the appearance of the sputum is**

A   purulent and scanty
B   frothy and blood-stained
C   mucopurulent and copious
D   mucoid and viscid

25. **Which of the following signs and symptoms often herald the onset of agranulocytosis:**

    A   sore throat and fever
    B   dizziness
    C   skeletal pain
    D   nausea and vomiting

26. **Which one of the following is a sign of acute left ventricular failure:**

    A   pulmonary oedema
    B   jugular venous congestion
    C   severe albuminuria
    D   pitting oedema of the legs

27. **The symptoms of pernicious anaemia do not usually appear until long after the onset of the disorder because**

    A   long-term supplies of vitamin B_{12} are stored in the liver
    B   long-term supplies of folic acid are stored in the liver
    C   vitamin B_{12} is manufactured by the liver
    D   folic acid is manufactured by the liver

28. **A self-employed man has angina pectoris in hospital. Which of the following would best allay his anxiety:**

    A   ask the doctor to prescribe diazepam
    B   allow him to have a little work to do
    C   tell him not to worry too much
    D   encourage him to discuss the worries

29. **Secondary haemorrhage after tonsillectomy is caused by**

    A   a slipped ligature
    B   eating hard sharp food
    C   infection
    D   a blood clot

30. **What is the most likely cause of excessive heat loss in the pre-term baby:**

    A   immature heat regulating system
    B   poor feeding reflex
    C   inadequate clothing or warmth
    D   reduced metabolism

31. **It is *most* important to allay pre-operative anxiety because it interferes with**

    A   sleeping and rest
    B   gastric emptying times
    C   co-operation and relaxation
    D   relationships with staff

32. **A young man who is a known epileptic has been admitted to the ward of which you are in charge. During the night, he has a grand mal seizure in his sleep. The following morning you should**

    A   keep him on strict bed rest for the day
    B   allow him to get up for toilet purposes only
    C   allow him to get up to watch television in the dayroom
    D   allow him to get up and encourage him to be active

33. **A patient is admitted for cataract extraction. Which of the following would lead to postponement of surgery pending further investigation:**

    A   frequency of micturition
    B   slight nocturnal confusion
    C   an irritating cough
    D   partial vision in the good eye

34. **A patient has a left-sided craniotomy. Which symptom would be reported immediately:**

    A   increasing right-sided weakness
    B   hypertension and bradycardia
    C   muscle twitching
    D   serous fluid oozing from the wound

35. **Following hypophysectomy a patient is likely to develop**

    A   diabetes mellitus
    B   renal failure
    C   liver failure
    D   diabetes insipidus

36. **The result of lack of thyroxine in a child is**

    A   normal stature, low mentality
    B   normal stature, normal mentality
    C   short stature, low mentality
    D   short stature, normal mentality

37. **A diabetic patient finds difficulty in injecting himself in the arm. He would find it best to inject the insulin into**

A   the flesh at the inside of his thighs
B   his buttock
C   the flesh of his abdomen
D   the flesh of his side

38. **After which of the following operations would it be *most* essential to record blood pressure:**

A   gastrectomy
B   adrenalectomy
C   panproctocolectomy
D   pneumonectomy

39. **An elderly patient is confused on the first night following admission. This is *most* likely to be due to**

A   cerebral anoxia
B   potassium deficiency
C   untreated anaemia
D   unfamiliar surroundings

40. **Which one of the following is most likely to pass undetected when a patient has a plaster cast in place:**

A   nerve injury
B   restricted circulation
C   wasting of the part
D   pressure sores

49. **A passive artificial immunity against measles is established with a dose of**

    A   measles toxoid
    B   anti-measles serum
    C   modified measles antigen
    D   measles immunoglobulins

50. **To effectively prevent pressure sore formation it is of *most* value to be aware of the**

    A   patient's protein and fluid intake
    B   length of time since the patient was last moved
    C   weight and drug regime of the patient
    D   criterion for identifying those patients at risk.

51. **Which one of the following results in local vasodilation:**

    A   adrenaline
    B   thromboplastin
    C   acetylcholine
    D   histamine

52. **The aim of first aid treatment of a superficial burn of the forearm is to**

    A   reduce heat and minimise the risk of infection
    B   reduce heat and prevent blisters forming
    C   clean the area and prevent blisters forming
    D   clean the area and minimise the risk of infection

53. Which one of the following is the antidote to heparin:

- A vitamin K
- B protamine sulphate
- C streptokinase
- D phenindione

54. Spironalatone antagonises

- A antidiuretic hormone secretion
- B aldosterone secretion
- C adrenaline secretion
- D renin secretion

55. Carbimazole affects the thyroid gland by

- A increasing its vascularity
- B reducing its size
- C inhibiting its uptake of iodine
- D reducing its vascularity

56. The process of cross-matching involves the matching of the

- A recipient's serum against the donor's red cells
- B donor's serum against the recipient's red cells
- C recipient's serum against the donor's serum
- D donor's red cells against the recipient's red cells

57. **The most useful treatment of hypertension is to give a drug which will**

   A   increase sympathetic and slow down parasympathetic activity
   B   decrease sympathetic and slow down parasympathetic activity
   C   decrease sympathetic and increase parasympathetic activity
   D   increase sympathetic and increase parasympathetic activity

58. **The most likely complications of a prolonged course of streptomycin are**

   A   tinnitus, vertigo, deafness and ataxia
   B   ataxia, deafness, rash and diarrhoea
   C   diarrhoea, rash, nausea and vomiting
   D   nausea, vomiting, tinnitus and vertigo

59. **Which one of the following incidents requires attention first:**

   A   a patient receiving blood transfusion develops rigors and complains of aches and pains
   B   an asthmatic patient becomes excited, distressed and breathless in an argument
   C   a diabetic patient looks pale and clammy and becomes increasingly drowsy
   D   the underwater seal drainage equipment of a pneumothorax patient stops swinging

60. **Which of the following should cause *most* concern. A patient receiving**

   A   gold injections develops albuminuria
   B   vincristine develops constipation
   C   cyclophosphamide develops alopecia
   D   prednisolone develops glycosuria

END OF PRACTICE EXAMINATION

PRACTICE EXAM ANSWERS

1. **C   61%**

   Officers of the General Nursing Council visit all training schools at regular intervals in order to ascertain that standards are being maintained. The syllabus of instruction, examinations, disciplinary matters and the maintenance of a Register and Roll of Nurses are part of the overall responsibility of the General Nursing Council.

2. **A   25%**

   The findings of this study are alarming and illustrate a lack of attention in both the preparation of and administration of nasogastric feeds to unconscious patients. It is a fundamental nursing activity to ensure that every patient has an adequate diet. This research shows that prescribing and administering nasogastric feeds were, in the hospitals studied, primarily a nursing responsibility.

3. **B   74%**

   Always consult the nurse in charge before answering telephone queries. It is possible that there may be some change regarding the patient of which you are not aware. It is impossible to confirm the enquirer's identity in this situation.

4. **B   45%**

   Before ten months, a baby does not normally have sufficient strength to stand on his own and his balance is unlikely to be sufficiently developed.

5. **B   44%**

   Swelling occurs following injury because permeability of the capillaries is increased, allowing fluid to escape into surrounding tissues. (Permeability means the degree to which fluid can pass from one structure to another through a wall or membrane).

6. **A 63%**

The newly admitted patient is in a state of mental conflict which commonly results in the patient remaining silent and introverted. The patient is in a constant condition of anxious expectation, characterised by fear and anxiety. This can also make the patient sensitive to noise and other external stimuli. Palpitations, nausea, indigestion, sweating and sleeplessness are also common features.

7. **C 62%**

A counselling session is a useful way of reducing emotional tension. Talking out the problem with a sympathetic listener who can remain objective, enables the person to resolve the problem and find a satisfactory solution in the majority of cases.

8. **A 59%**

When the right ventricle fails, the pressure rises in the right atrium, vena cava, the hepatic and the systemic veins. The effects of systemic venous congestion are engorged veins, enlarged and tender liver and oedema can be easily observed. Oedema is a valuable sign of right heart failure and is best seen in the dependent parts, the feet when upright and the backs of the thighs and lumbar region when in bed.

9. **D 67%**

Carbon monoxide is a colourless poisonous gas formed by burning carbon or organic fuels with a scanty supply of oxygen. It causes asphyxiation by combining irreversibly with the blood haemoglobin. This substance circulating in the capillaries gives the cherry red appearance.

10. **B 71%**

Always face deaf patients when speaking to them — facial expression aids understanding as well as clear lip movement.

11. **C   64%**

    The reason for administering low percentage oxygen to a patient with an acute exacerbation of chronic bronchitis is to maintain respiratory function by anoxic response. Usually, long continued carbon dioxide retention leads to failure in response of the respiratory centre to a rise in the carbon dioxide content of the blood. In these circumstances, high concentration of oxygen may diminish ventilation and produce first depressed respiration and finally apnoea. The result will be increasing carbon dioxide retention and deterioration of the condition of the patient.

12. **B   49%**

    In bronchiectasis, physiotherapy (in particular postural drainage) is a very important principle. If bronchial secretions are expelled, the danger of infection is minimised and antibiotics may not be required.

13. **A   63%**

    Coeliac disease is thought to be an allergic reaction. The culprit is gluten, and the first principle of treatment is to remove gluten from the diet.
    An effort must be made to adhere to a gluten-free diet.

14. **B   36%**

    Removal of the terminal ilium can result in pernicious anaemia through loss of the absorption of vitamin B_{12}. This can be prevented by giving injections of vitamin B_{12} (cyanocobalamin) in doses of 100-1000 micrograms intramuscularly.

15. **A   71%**

    Raised pressure in the portal vein can lead to oesophageal varices. In this condition the veins at the lower end of the oesophagus, where the portal veins anastomose with those of the general circulation, become dilated and varicose. They may rupture and the escaping blood is subsequently vomited.

16.   **D   37%**

The sphincter of Oddi controls the flow of bile into the duodenum.
Bile contains bile pigments and these will be present in excess in the blood. In turn, these pigments will escape into the tissues including the skin, giving it a yellow colour. This form of jaundice is called obstructive jaundice. If no bile pigments reach the intestines, the stools lose their characteristic brown colour and become clay coloured (steatorrhoea). Some of the excess bile pigments circulating in the blood will be excreted in the urine, which will become very dark in colour.

17.   **B   70%**

If a patient is dying, it is kinder and more humane to let the patient have a bottle of beer as requested. This will not interfere with the ultimate outcome of the disease, but will make the patient's last days more bearable if not carried to excess.

18.   **B   74%**

The repair of an umbilical hernia should not interfere with micturition.
The elderly lady may be a little drowsy following surgery, she may be confused, disorientated, or in pain. She may also feel uncomfortable and embarrassed about using a bedpan, so she needs time and privacy to prevent retention of urine. Turning the taps on will help.

19.   **B   76%**

The peritoneal membrane is a semi-permeable membrane and if dialysing fluid is introduced via a catheter into the cavity, it will cause electrolytes and metabolic waste to move from the body into the peritoneal cavity by osmosis and diffusion.

20.   **C   74%**

Protein loss in nephrotic syndrome is very significant and is detected as severe albuminuria. Albumin, the largest fraction of the plasma proteins, is not normally filtered from the blood by the renal glomerulus — its molecular size is too large for filtration. Where the kidney is damaged, however, albumin is lost in quantity and must be replaced.

21. D 33%

If the plasma level of a substance exceeds the renal threshold for that substance, the kidneys will excrete the substance into the urine until the plasma level returns to normal.

22. A 41%

Cutting the child's finger nails is considered most important because the ova of the female threadworm are laid around the anus where intense itching occurs, especially at night. The child's fingers may then carry the ova to the mouth causing re-infection.

23. A 80%

Central venous pressure may be measured by introducing a fine catheter via a major vein into the superior vena cava, into the right atrium. The pressure in the right atrium may then be measured. The normal range is 4-10 cm of water.

24. B 55%

In left ventricular failure, the sputum is bloodstained and aereated, causing frothing.

25. A 74%

Agranulocytosis is lack of white blood cells. As the function of white blood cells is protection against infection, the first most commonly affected areas are mucous membrane and broken skin. So the patient develops a sore throat and consequent infection producing a fever. Other symptoms are malaise, rapid weak pulse, dysphagia, ulcers on oral mucosa and ulceration of the pharynx.

26. **A   64%**

Pulmonary oedema is the widespread exudation or transudation of liquid into the alveolar walls and spaces, from the pulmonary capillaries. A rise in the pulmonary capillary pressure due to left ventricular failure, mitral valve disease and pulmonary veno-occlusive disease is by the far the commonest cause of pulmonary oedema. Breathlessness is the outstanding symptom and may be extremely distressing.

27. **A   70%**

Anaemia implies some deficiency in the quality or in the quantity of the blood. In pernicious anaemia, lack of the intrinsic factor makes it impossible for vitamin B_{12} to be absorbed. Long-term supplies of vitamin B_{12} are stored in the liver so until these are exhausted, symptoms do not present.

28. **D   64%**

Discussion of the problem would allay anxiety because to talk over the problem with a sympathetic listener reduces anxiety levels. Some physiological changes which occur in anxiety are tachycardia, sweating and tremor. These signs and symptoms can be noted by the nurse attending the patient.

29. **C   69%**

Secondary haemorrhage can only be caused by infection. This is usually around ten days after the operation. Slipped ligature, eating hard food and a blood clot are likely to cause reactionary haemorrhage, occurring some hours after surgery.

30. **A   72%**

In the immature infant the heat regulating centre in the brain is not fully functional. While the baby is within the mother's womb it is in a perfectly controlled environmental temperature and the heat regulating centre is not required to function. This leads to problems for the pre-term (premature) baby becuase there can be excessive heat loss due to the fact that the heat regulating centre does not respond to the changing environmental temperature.

31. **B** 43%

Whilst anxiety will interfere with A B C and D to some degree, it is *most* important to remember that gastric emptying time could be delayed, contributing to post-operative vomiting and attendant risks.

32. **D** 51%

Epilepsy is a condition in which disturbance of the cerebral cortex produces convulsive movements, which in the case of grand mal seizures are accompanied by unconsciousness and often incontinence. It is important to be aware of the patient's behaviour after the seizure; however, once the mental condition has returned to normal, then the patient should be encouraged to do as much for himself as possible. The nurse must always be aware of the patient's activities and whereabouts, so as not to leave him in a potential dangerous situation such as alone in the bathroom.

33. **C** 69%

An irritating cough could cause complications after cataract extraction because of the violent movement of the patient's head induced by the cough, and the raised pressure within the cranial cavity.

34. **B** 40%

The *most* important observations to report are hypertension and bradycardia as these are signs of increasing intra-cranial pressure. This increase in pressure may be due to the actual brain tissue swelling or be due to haemorrhage within the cranium. Other observations need also be reported as damage to the left side of the brain will affect the right side of the body. Muscular twitching is a sign of abnormal electrical conduction in the brain and needs to be controlled. Serous fluid oozing from the wound could indicate infection.

35. **D** 53%

Diabetes insipidus is likely to develop after hypophysectomy because the antidiuretic hormone secreted by the pituitary is absent. This results in large quantities of pale coloured urine with a low specific gravity being passed.

36. C 71%

Cretinism is a congenital disorder caused by lack of thyroxine.
Stunted growth and mental impairment results.

37. C 70%

Insulin is administered as a subcutaneous injection. The sites used
in the body for subcutaneous injections are the upper, outer
aspects of the arm, the abdomen or the upper outer aspect of the
thighs.

38. B 68%

One of the complications of adrenalectomy is a low blood
pressure. If the patient does become hypotensive, then the dosage
and/or frequency of hydrocortisone must be increased.

39. D 72%

Elderly patients are likely to become confused if they wake up
during the night and find themselves in a strange environment.
This is the *most* likely cause of confusion on the first night
following admission.

40. C 37%

This is because the part is obscured by the plaster cast. In some
cases, it can be detected by the plaster cast becoming more
movable on the affected limb and loose fitting because of the
wastage of muscle tissue due to lack of exercise.

41.   C   72%

A fat embolism may complicate a fracture. If a portion of fat from the bone marrow passes into a torn vein and circulates in the bloodstream, it could cause fatal cerebral consequences. Fortunately, it is rare.

42.   D   68%

As the urethra is close to the anterior vaginal wall, it is likely to become bruised during surgery which, with attendant swelling, can lead to retention. A catheter is left in place post-operatively to help prevent this.

43.   C   65%

When a graafian follicle reaches the surface of the ovary it ruptures, and the ovum and the follicular fluid it contains escapes. A group of cells form and fills the cavity of the follicle. These cells are characteristically yellow and are called the luteal (yellow) cells. Blood capillaries grow into the mass of cells and thus the corpus luteum is formed. Luteinising hormone assists the follicle stimulating hormone to promote follicular ripening.

44.   A   33%

In vaginal prolapse, the vagina drops down, dragging with it the uterus. The vaginal walls are stretched so that the bladder bulges into the anterior wall. The commonest cause is childbearing, but general ill-health combined with overwork and fatigue (contributing to poor muscle tone and atrophy of the uterine ligaments) can also contribute. Micturition may be frequent and difficult.

45.   A   56%

Intra-uterine contraceptive devices prevent conception by preventing the fertilised ovum becoming implanted. They can cause menstrual upsets, dysmenorrhoea, pelvic infections and pregnancy can occur with them in place. It is therefore recommended that they are used with a spermicidal agent.

46. D 42%

Triple immunisation protects against tetanus, whooping cough and diphtheria, given when the child is aged 3 months, 4 months, 5 months and 17 months. Diphtheria vaccine and tetanus toxoid are repeated at 4½ years. Polio vaccine is given separately at ages 3 months, 4 months, 5 months and 4½ years.

47. B 67%

The hypersensitive reaction to an antigen is caused by a release of histamine in the tissues. Antigens may be soluble substances such as toxins and foreign proteins or bacteria and tissue cells.

48. C 73%

Reverse barrier nursing is the term used to describe the nursing technique by which a patient who is vulnerable to infection, e.g. burns, transplant patients, is prevented from acquiring any infection. This necessitates strict isolation of the patient and competent barrier nursing to prevent any micro-organisms coming into contact with the patient. It is called reverse barrier nursing because the aim is to prevent bacteria gaining access to the patient. In normal barrier nursing, the nursing technique is to prevent organisms from the patient coming into contact with other individuals.

49. C 44%

Modified measles antigen produces passive acquired immunity in the individual receiving it. It is quick-acting but of relatively short duration in its action. Passive immunity is the conferral of specific immunity on previously non-immune individuals by the administration of sensitized lymphoid cells or serum from immune individuals.

50. D 36%

Whilst A B and C are all factors to be considered, it would be *most* useful if nursing staff were able to identify patients at risk and initiate preventative measures. The "Norton scale" is of great value in such identification.

51.   D   44%

Histamine is a substance contained in the tissues of the body, particularly in the skin and intestinal tract. It is released on injury to the tissues or on the injection of a foreign protein. It causes vasodilatation of the blood vessels.

52.   A   74%

The first aid treatment for a superficial burn on the forearm is to immerse it in cold water, after removing any obstacles such as clothing, watch or jewellery, and then to cover it with a clean dressing. This treatment is given to reduce the heat and minimize the risk of infection. Blisters will form depending on the depth of the skin burn. Reducing the heat also reduces the pain the patient is experiencing.

53.   B   71%

Protamine sulphate is the antidote to heparin. Each distractor A, C and D are linked in some way to the blood clotting process, hence their inclusion as alternative answers.
A) vitamin K is essential for effective blood clotting
C) streptokinase is an enzyme used to liquify clotted blood
D) phenindione (the proprietary name for Dindevan) is an orally active anticoagulant.

54.   B   49%

Spironalactone antagonises the secretion of aldosterone, therefore reabsorption of sodium in the renal tubule is impaired. Because of this, the sodium is excreted in the urine attracting extra water with it, and diuresis is improved.

55.   C   57%

Carbimazole has the effect of depressing the formation of thyroxine and inhibiting uptake of iodine by the gland. Minor side effects include headache, rash and gastric upset.

56.   A   29%

The process of cross matching involves matching the *recipient's serum* against the *donor red cells*. The agglutinins present in the recipient's serum will react against specific agglutinogens on the donor's red cell. If agglutination occurs, the donor blood cannot be given to the recipient.

57.   C   45%

The control of blood pressure is partly affected by the relative balance of the sympathetic and parasympathetic nervous systems. Drugs which will inhibit the sympathetic nervous system, causing vasodilatation, have the effect of lowering the blood pressure.

58.   A   34%

Streptomycin is notoriously ototoxic. The exact reasons for this are as yet unknown, but hearing and balance may well become involved. Hence, tinnitus, vertigo, deafness and ataxia are regarded as complications of streptomycin therapy.

59.   C   57%

A diabetic who looks pale with a clammy skin and becoming increasingly drowsy, signifies that the patient is developing hypoglycaemia. This is characterised by an abnormally low blood sugar and causes marked alteration of the nervous system. It is essential that glucose in water is given to the patient to drink before consciousness is lost.

60.   A   35%

Gold preparations are given with great caution and it is important to watch for toxic symptoms such as albuminuria, rise in temperature, skin rashes, urticaria and gastrointestinal disturbance.

End of Practice Exam Answers